MORE EVERYDAY AIDS
AND APPLIANCES

MORE
EVERYDAY AIDS
AND APPLIANCES

Edited by

GRAHAM MULLEY, FRCP

Professor, Department of Medicine for the Elderly
St James's University Hospital, Leeds

Articles from the *British Medical Journal*

Published by the British Medical Journal
Tavistock Square, London WC1H 9JR

First published 1991

British Library Cataloguing in Publication Data

More everyday aids and appliances.
  I. Mulley, Graham P, *(Graham Peter)*
362.4028

ISBN 0–7279–0283–0

Typeset and printed in Great Britain by
Latimer Trend & Co Ltd, Plymouth

Contents

Appliances

Mobility aids

Introduction

Do you know how to remove a patient's artificial eye and clean it? Can you confidently advise on the management of dentures or how to take care of a wig? Do you know whom to refer for splints or callipers? Or how to provide a blind person with a guide dog? This book of articles reprinted from the *British Medical Journal* will help you with these and many other practical problems encountered by disabled patients.

The challenge of rehabilitation is to restore disabled people to their optimum levels of independence and wellbeing. This is achieved in a number of ways: sustaining morale and motivation; preventing or mitigating the physical and psychological complications of illness; deploying specialised techniques; supplying personal help; and providing enabling equipment and compensatory appliances. Aids should therefore be provided only after a detailed assessment of the individual. This will usually involve close communication between doctors, therapists, nurses, and other professionals, and between health workers and patients and their families.

In many cases the use of gadgets can be obviated by learning alternative ways of performing everyday activities (sliding heavy pans rather than lifting them; wearing modified clothing so that independence can be maintained). When aids are indicated it is often the simple ones that are most used and most useful—shoehorns, grab rails, handrails on staircases, large dials on telephones, blocks to raise beds to the optimum height, modified car key handles.

We all need to move. One section of the book is devoted entirely to mobility aids: those items which can help someone climb and descend stairs; ramps, the provision of which might allow many housebound people to go outside; modified car controls, which enable disabled drivers to have greater freedom of mobility. Specialised mobility aids for disabled children are considered, as are crutches, which are mainly used by young and middle aged adults. Walking frames are used predominantly by those elderly people who have difficulty in balancing. If they do fall both they and their families will feel reassured if an emergency alarm is available.

Prostheses are appliances which help to compensate for a missing or non-functioning part of the body. The loss of a breast or eye, teeth or hair can cause psychological problems which need careful consideration. The prompt and sensitive provision of acceptable appliances can do much to improve the lives of those who feel embarrassed or depressed by their loss.

Orthoses support or correct the function of a deficient limb or organ. The varieties of splints and callipers are considered here.

Aids that encourage people to perform everyday tasks are also discussed. A greater awareness of dressing, feeding, and kitchen aids may result in more people being referred to occupational therapists for assessment.

Disabled people like to have fun, just as able bodied people do, and equipment and opportunities for leisure activities are reviewed.

We also consider aids that help in nursing patients in bed: not only the range of bed aids but also low pressure surfaces, which can do so much to prevent painful and unsightly pressure sores.

I am grateful to the contributors, who have all written interesting and straightforward accounts of which aids are available, how to get them, how much they cost, what complications they may cause, and where to obtain further advice and information. I am sure that you will find these chapters useful, and I hope that you enjoy reading the book as much as I have enjoyed editing it.

GRAHAM MULLEY

Aids to home care

Aids for visual impairment

N J DUDLEY

Introduction

The World Health Organisation has proposed that a visual acuity of less than 6/18 on a Snellen chart is a suitable definition of visual impairment. Anyone with such a degree of impairment should be seen by an ophthalmologist to exclude treatable eye disease. People with severe visual impairment may then be registered as blind or partially sighted.

Registration as blind is defined by the National Assistance Act of 1948 as "so blind as to be unable to perform any work for which sight is essential": a visual acuity either below 3/60 or one of 3/60 but less than 6/60 if the field of vision is considerably contracted or 6/60 or above if the field of vision is very contracted. There is no statutory definition for partial sight but guidelines imply that the person registered is "substantially and permanently handicapped." For registration purposes this means a visual acuity of either 3/60 to 6/60 with a full field, or up to 6/24 with a moderate field constriction, or 6/18 or even better if there is a gross field defect or definite constriction of the field.

The latest available figures show that in 1988 just over a quarter of a million people in England, Scotland, and Wales were registered as blind or partially sighted (table I). This represents 0·43% of the population and is likely to be an underestimate of those eligible for registration. The Royal National Institute for the Blind (RNIB) estimated from the findings of a recent government sponsored survey[1] that no fewer than 960 000 people have a sight defect so severe that they should be registered as blind or partially sighted.[2] Severe visual impairment affects mostly elderly people: in

3

TABLE I—Number of people registered as blind or partially sighted in 1988

	Registered blind	Registered partially sighted	Population
England	126 828	79 048	47 536 300
Scotland	13 760	4 651	5 094 000
Wales	8 564	5 764	2 857 031
Total	149 152	89 463	55 487 331

Figures from Department of Health, Scottish Office, Welsh Office, and Office of Population Censuses and Surveys.

TABLE II—Registered blind or partially sighted population in England in 1988. Percentages supplied by Department of Health

Age (years)	Registered blind (% of total registered blind)	Registered partially sighted (% of total registered partially sighted)
0·4	0·4	0·3
5–15	1·3	2·1
16–49	10·2	13·0
50–64	9·9	8·5
65–74	15·4	14·9
≥75	63·0	61·1

England nearly four fifths of people registered as blind and over three quarters of people registered as partially sighted are over 65 (table II). The commonest conditions causing visual impairment are cataract, macular degeneration, glaucoma, and diabetic retinopathy.

Social services

Registration as blind or partially sighted is important as it brings the patient to the attention of the local authority social services, who can arrange a visit by a social worker, preferably one trained in dealing with the problems of the visually disabled, to assess the needs of each newly registered client. The social services has a legal obligation to look after the welfare of blind and partially sighted people and should be able to provide rehabilitation courses in the activities of daily living, teach new communication skills such as braille, and provide mobility training. Unfortunately, these services are not taken up by most elderly registered people. Aids can be offered by the social services, finances permitting; those commonly offered are writing aids, talking books, liquid level indicators, big button phones and phone dial adaptations, talking clocks, and symbol canes. Only those people registered as blind are entitled to a free radio or cassette player.

Reading and writing aids

There are many people who are neither blind nor partially sighted but have such a degree of visual impairment that their near visual acuity is not good enough to read normal size print in newspapers, magazines, or books. Increasing the size of the print allows some people to read without the need for any special aids and nowadays most public libraries have a selection of books in large print. Newspapers and magazines do not usually have large print editions and the visually impaired reader therefore has to use a low vision aid (fig 1) to read them. Low vision aids can be obtained on free loan from hospital eye clinics.[3]

For those who are unable to read books the RNIB provides a valuable service. The Talking Book Service has some 70 000 members and about 8000 titles to choose from. Membership is open to anyone who has a near visual acuity with their normal reading glasses of N12 or less (fig 2). The talking book cassettes can be played only on a talking book machine, which is supplied on free loan by the RNIB. There is a fee for membership of this service. The RNIB also has an extensive cassette library containing some 10 000 non-fiction titles, mainly academic books, recorded on C90 cassettes. Conditions for membership of the cassette library are the same as for the talking book library.

There are two systems of embossed script for reading and writing: braille and moon. Louis Braille invented the first system in 1824; its symbols are made up of variations of up to six raised dots arranged in a domino six pattern. The symbols in Dr William Moon's system are based on the roman alphabet. Few blind people are able to read either system. Details of books and magazines published by the RNIB in both systems can be obtained from the RNIB Customer Services at Peterborough.

There are now reading machines that can convert print into

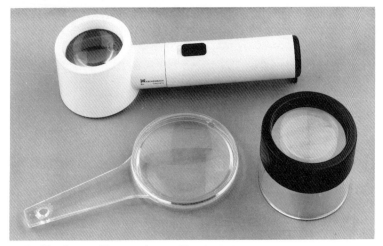

FIG 1—Simple magnifiers: torch magnifier (*back*), hand magnifier (*front left*), desk magnifier (*front right*)

You can join the Talking Book Library if your vision is certified as N12 or less. If you cannot read this paragraph wearing your normal reading glasses, you probably qualify for membership.

FIG 2—Eligibility for membership of RNIB's Talking Book Service. (Reproduced courtesy of RNIB)

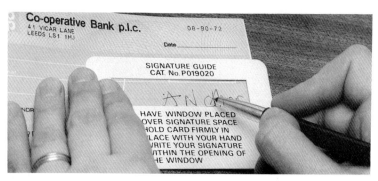

FIG 3—Signature guide

synthetic speech, braille, or a tactile form. The main disadvantages of these machines are that they are very expensive and not widely available.

A variety of writing aids is obtainable from the RNIB to help with signatures, writing cheques, addressing envelopes, and letter writing. The first three aids are pieces of either plastic or cardboard with windows for writing on the underlying paper (figs 3 and 4). For letter writing there is a choice of six writing frames to help the user write in straight, parallel lines (fig 5). Alternatives are paper embossed with horizontal lines, available from the RNIB, or writing paper with heavy lines, available from the Partially Sighted Society.

Kitchen aids

In the London showroom of the Disabled Living Foundation there is a permanent display kitchen featuring over 200 aids for the visually impaired cook. Most have not been designed specifically for people with impaired vision and can be bought from high street shops. A catalogue of items on display can be obtained from the Disabled Living Foundation.

It is often the simple aids that are the most useful, such as the liquid level indicator, a cylindrical device from which two pairs of plastic covered prongs protrude: one short, the other long (fig 6). The device is hooked over the edge of a cup by one of the pairs of prongs and when the liquid makes contact it makes an audible signal. It has been modified for deaf–blind people so that it vibrates on contact with liquid. Another aid with many uses is Hi-marks, a bright orange paste that is squeezed out of a tube through a fine nozzle. When it sets it forms a highly visible and tactile marking. It adheres to metal, plastic, paper, and fabrics and can be used, for example, to mark the controls of cookers, microwaves, irons, etc, and to label containers or clothing. Other useful kitchen aids are the Dux slicing knife, which has an adjustable guard to vary the slice width, and the Flasher electronic gas lighter, which is safer and easier to use than matches.

Telephone aids

Telephones present a problem for the visually impaired person as the numbers on the old style phones and the numbers and

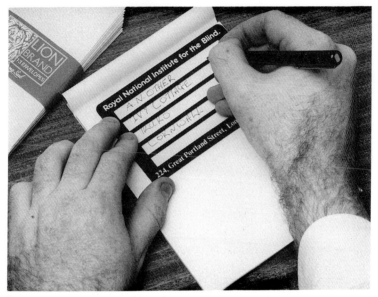

FIG 4—Envelope address guide

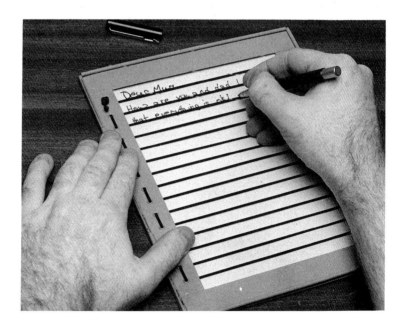

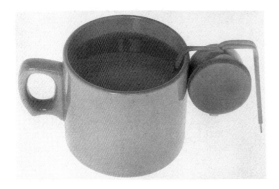

FIG 6—Liquid level indicator

buttons on the new pushbutton phones are too small to be clearly seen. British Telecom can supply free of charge an enlarged numeral dial ring, which has large black numbers on a white background, to stick on the phone (fig 7). The second problem is overcome by pushbutton phones with big buttons. Two suitable models are the Audioline 310, available from British Telecom shops, and the Dialatron Big Button phone (fig 8), and they can be purchased from the Partially Sighted Society in a modified form with 2·5 cm black numbers on a white background and operating instructions in large print. Further information on equipment and services for the visually impaired can be found in British Telecom's *Guide to Equipment and Services for Disabled Customers*.

Watches and clocks

The RNIB stocks three types of watch and a range of clocks. There is an "easy to see watch," designed for people with some useful residual vision, which has large black numerals with black hands on a white background and comes in 2·5 cm and 3 cm diameters. A talking watch is available, as are tactile watches, which have hinged glass fronts, raised dots to mark the hours, and strengthened hands. Kitchen clocks with large numerals can be bought from high street shops to be used by those with residual vision. Smaller tactile clocks and a talking clock (fig 9) can be purchased from the RNIB.

9

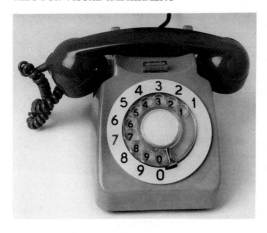

FIG 7—Enlarged numeral dial fitted to standard dial phone

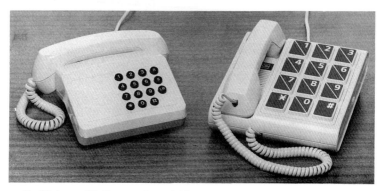

FIG 8—Dialatron Big Button phone (*right*) compared with standard push button phone (*left*)

Mobility aids

The most commonly used mobility aids are canes, sticks, and guide dogs. Canes come in three varieties: symbol canes, guide canes, and long canes (fig 10). Strictly speaking, a symbol cane is not a mobility aid (it is used to indicate that the person holding the cane has a visual disability), but it is useful as a probe or buffer. Guide canes and long canes are true mobility aids and require instruction in their use by a mobility instructor, especially for the long cane, which was developed in the 1940s to aid the rehabilitation of second world war veterans. The cane is swung in an arc in

10

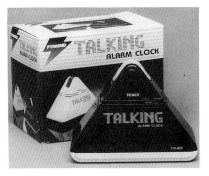

FIG 9—Pyramid talking clock

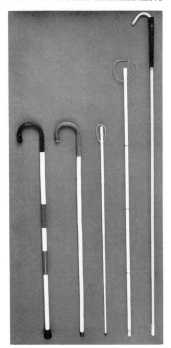

FIG 10—Mobility aids (*left to right*) red and white banded stick, white stick, symbol cane, guide cane, long cane

front of the body and allows changes in ground level and obstructions below waist height to be detected. With these aids fairly rapid and safe mobility can be achieved.

Canes are not designed to provide support for the user. If this is needed then a white stick made of wood or aluminium should be used. Canes and sticks banded with red tape indicate that the user has a hearing impairment as well. All sticks and canes are available from the RNIB.

Guide dogs are provided by the Guide Dogs for the Blind Association, which welcomes applications for a guide dog from any registered blind person aged over 16 living in the United Kingdom who is fit enough to be able to use and care for a dog. An application may be made by the blind person or by someone acting on his or her behalf to any of the training centres or the main headquarters in Windsor. There are currently 11 training centres around the country. The association is trying to increase the amount of domiciliary training because a long period away from home on a residential training course may be unacceptable to

11

potential trainees. There are about 4000 working guide dogs, and 597 new guide dogs were supplied in 1988, almost a sixth of them to people over the age of 65. Although guide dogs are excellent aids to mobility they are in relatively short supply and are available to less than 3% of registered blind people.

Summary

This chapter provides only a flavour of the type and range of aids available to the visually impaired person. Many other aids for leisure, learning, and daily living are illustrated in the RNIB equipment and games catalogue.

1 Office of Population Censuses and Surveys. *Survey of disability in Great Britain. Report 1. The prevalence of disability among adults.* London: HMSO, 1988.
2 Royal National Institute for the Blind. *Report for the year ended 31st March 1989.* London: RNIB, 1989.
3 Hillman JS. Aids for low vision in the elderly. *BMJ* 1988,**296**:102-3.

Appendix

Useful addresses

Royal National Institute for the Blind, 224 Great Portland Street, London W1N 6AA (071 388 1266)

RNIB Customer Services, Production and Distribution Centre, Bakewell Road, Orton, Southgate, Peterborough PE2 0XU (0733 370777)

RNIB Talking Book Service, Mount Pleasant, Alperton, Wembley, Middlesex HA0 1RR

The Guide Dogs for the Blind Association, Head Office, Alexandra House, Park Street, Windsor, Berkshire SL4 1JR (0753 855711)

Partially Sighted Society, Queens Road, Doncaster DN1 2NX (0302 323132)

Disabled Living Foundation, 380/384 Harrow Road, London W9 2HU (071 289 6111). The Disabled Living Foundation will provide the address of your local Disabled Living Centre, which provides helpful advice on equipment for disability.

Further reading

British Broadcasting Corporation. *The in touch handbook.* Available from Broadcasting Support Services, PO Box 7, London W3 6XJ (Price £8.50)

Ford M. *In touch at home.* Available from ISIS, 55 St Thomas's Street, Oxford OX1 1JG (Price £5.95)

Royal National Institute for the Blind. *Equipment and games catalogue.* Available from RNIB, Customer Services (address above)

British Telecom. *Guide to equipment and services for disabled customers.* Available free from British Telecom shops.

Aids to prevent pressure sores

JOHN B YOUNG

Pressure sores are a potentially preventable complication of immobilising illnesses. They can be painful and distressing to the patient and may necessitate long periods in hospital. They are expensive: treatment of pressure sores costs the NHS an estimated £150 million a year.[1] Although treatment of the established sore is important, methods of prevention should be our main concern. Vulnerable patients must be identified and appropriate nursing methods and equipment selected. I have concentrated mainly on beds and mattresses, but all surfaces on which patients sit or lie, including easy chairs, wheelchairs, casualty trolleys, and operating tables,[2] need attention.

Mechanisms of pressure sore formation

Pressure sores originate deep within subcutaneous tissues. The body can withstand high pressures if uniformly applied (such as for deep sea divers) but local (point) pressure and shearing forces produce tissue distortion and so impair or occlude capillary flow producing ischaemia (fig 1). The standard NHS hospital mattress can produce point pressures of up to 150 mm Hg. Ischaemia is likely to develop if the normal capillary pressure of 12–33 mm Hg is exceeded for long enough. Critical capillary pressures may be lower in debilitated or elderly patients. Friction, a component of shear, may contribute separately to pressure sores by stripping superficial skin layers, leading to ulceration.

Preventing pressure sores

Prevention begins with good nursing care. Attention to hydration, nutrition, and skin care are important, and regular fre-

13

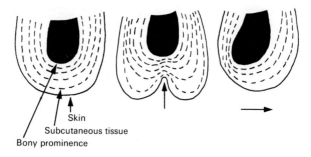

Skin
Subcutaneous tissue
Bony prominence

FIG 1—Unstressed subcutaneous tissue (*left*); deforming effects of point pressure (*centre*); and shear (*right*)

Norton score, for assessing degree of risk of developing pressure sores, developed for use with elderly patients. Score of ≤14 indicates vulnerability to pressure sores and score of <12 high risk

Physical condition	Mental state	Activity	Mobility	Incontinence
Good (4)	Alert (4)	Ambulant (4)	Full (4)	None (4)
Fair (3)	Apathetic (3)	Walks with help (3)	Slightly limited (3)	Occasional (3)
Poor (2)	Confused (2)	Chairbound (2)	Very limited (2)	Usually urine (2)
Very bad (1)	Stuporous (1)	Bedbound (1)	Immobile (1)	Double (1)

quent turning will restore subcutaneous perfusion. These measures are enough for most patients but patients at high risk of pressure sores also require special pressure relieving surfaces. High risk patients should be identified by routine use of one of the available prediction scales[3]—for example, the Norton score (table). In general, elderly patients and patients who have impaired consciousness or who are bed or chair bound, especially if spontaneous movement is reduced,[4] are most at risk.[5]

Pressure relieving surfaces

The dominant principle is that the supporting medium should mould around the body, providing equal pressure over the largest possible areas thereby eliminating point pressures and tissue

14

distortion. There needs to be enough depth so that the bony prominences do not "ground" on to the hard mattress base. Realising that the most advanced pressure relieving devices can be seriously undermined by tightly tucked in bedding, which produces a "hammock" effect with concomitant high pressure, is also important. Selecting a pressure relieving surface primarily entails an understanding of the degree of protection that a particular surface will provide. Other considerations are ease of use and maintenance, ease of nursing procedures including moving and transferring patients, patient acceptability, and cost.

Supplements to standard mattresses

The pressure relieving characteristics of the standard NHS mattress, especially when covered by a waterproof sheet, are poor and can be improved by a range of additional products. Sheepskin fleeces can be used to reduce shear and to improve vapour loss, which helps keep the skin dry. Natural fleeces are considerably better at both these functions than synthetic products,[6] but are more expensive (about £18 compared with £10). The physical properties of any type of fleece are impaired when overlaid by sheets or clothing and if matting occurs due to poor laundering. Various types of bootee are available to protect the heels, which are a particularly vulnerable site for pressure sores in elderly patients with a fractured neck of a femur. A gel pad cushion has proved effective for protecting the sacrum, even during traction.[7]

Padding mattresses (fig 2) containing polyester fibres (for example, Spenco or Polycare) laid on top of a standard mattress are probably as effective as ripple mattresses, especially for elderly people, but confer only a modest degree of extra protection and should not therefore be relied on for those patients judged to be at considerable risk of pressure sores.[8] They are easier to use than ripple mattresses and are maintenance free but should be replaced after two to three years. Also of proved effectiveness is a polystyrene bead bed system for use on trolleys and theatre tables as well as hospital mattresses.[9] It produces an instant three dimensional mould of the body contours so reducing point pressure and tissue deformation.

Foam mattresses

The Vaperm is the best studied mattress in this group. It is constructed from five types of fatigue resistant polyethylene foams

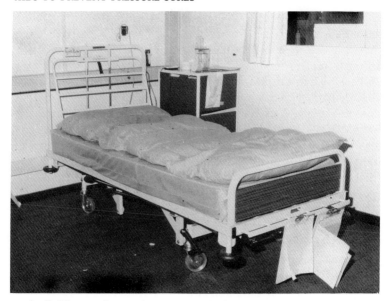

FIG 2—Padding overlay supplement to standard mattress; confers only modest degree of extra protection

each of varying densities laid together with pressure relieving and ventilation channels to produce a composite structure. The primary mattress cover is a thin washable or disposable polyurethane film that readily conforms to body indentations and is also waterproof but vapour permeable so preventing excessive skin moisture. This mattress is fairly cheap (£135), particularly when it is compared with a standard NHS mattress plus a padding supplement mattress or ripple mattress. Use and maintenance is also easy. Adequate ventilation requires an open mesh bed base—not the solid sheet of the King's Fund bed. The pressure relieving characteristics are considerably superior to those of the standard hospital foam mattress.[1]

Ripple mattresses

Ripple mattresses consist of tubular air filled cells, each of which is alternately inflated and deflated. Critical tissue ischaemia is therefore prevented by the vulnerable body pressure points being subjected to alternating short periods of high and low pressures. It is laid on to the standard mattress and connected to a pump unit and time switch. Several types of ripple mattress are available, but those with larger diameter cells (10 cm) are better as the smaller (5 cm) cells do not provide adquate support and may allow "grounding" to occur. This factor probably excludes the use of the even smaller "bubble pad" mattresses for which there is no proof of effectiveness.

The large cell ripple mattress is simple and effective,[10] but use has been marred by poor reliability.[11] In a recent study 45 ripple mattresses required 50 repairs of motors and 90 repairs of material during 12 months.[8] Constant vigilance and a routine maintenance programme are essential to ensure correct functioning. If the cells fail to deflate constant high tissue pressures occur thereby increasing the risk of pressure sores. A simple check is to ensure it is possible to reach under the patient via the deflated cell. Failure of the red warning light on the motor unit to go off indicates low pressure and a probable puncture. The tubing coil leading to the motor is easily kinked or obstructed, again causing malfunctioning of the mattress.

Airwave system

This is a more complex air cell type bed (fig 3). It has two layers of air cells rather than one, which are laid together as vertical pairs so providing up to 20 cm depth. Pressure is alternated by deflating every third cell in turn, each cycle lasting seven and a half minutes. The power unit is fairly quiet and easy to operate with the pressure set automatically and an audible malfunction alarm. In use the air cell mattress is simply laid on to a standard hospital bed base. The spaces left by the deflated cells make easy access for lifting and turning the patient. The large cell diameter enables the patient to sit semirecumbent without excessive shearing forces on the buttocks. The system is considerably more effective than a large cell ripple bed,[12] more robust and reliable, but is 20 times more expensive (£2350).

Air support systems (fig 4)

These are expensive and complex pressure relieving systems (£7450). High point pressures are avoided by supporting the patient on rows of transversely arranged microporous air sacs mounted on an integral bed frame that contains the air supply unit and heater. The sacs are arranged in sections that can be separately controlled. The sacs are waterproof but vapour permeable and air

17

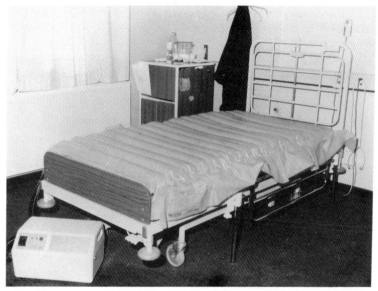

FIG 3—Airwave system (Pegasus): easy to use and suitable for high risk patients

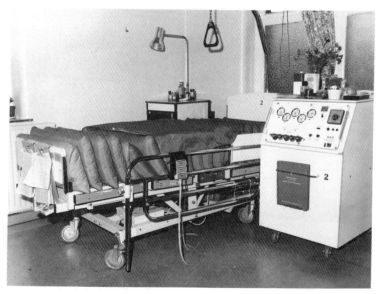

FIG 4—Low air loss bed (Mediscus): used for high risk patients in special departments such as intensive care

is continuously circulated through the perforations, which maintains a dry skin. Very low point pressures are achieved.[13] Weekly routine maintenance is required and a period of training needed to use this system effectively. The equipment is bulky, rather noisy, and probably best reserved for special cases such as intensive care and burns units.

Flotation beds

True flotation produces no pressure gradients and therefore no tissue distortion. Unfortunately, only deep tank systems can provide genuine flotation, and these are disadvantaged by cost, weight, and complexity of use. Shallow water beds inevitably cause some distortion through tension in the covering material or "grounding," or both. Whether they have any advantages over more manageable static or air mattresses is doubtful. All types of water bed have potential difficulties with regulating water temperature, restricting the patient's movement, and motion sickness in susceptible people. Moreover, nursing procedures on the unstable surface (especially lifting or transferring heavy or disabled patients) are awkward and special instruction is needed.

Dry flotation

Some of the disadvantages of water beds are overcome by "dry flotation" systems. Here the patient lies on a tank of glass microspheres that are converted into a "fluid" medium by blowing air through them. The flotation instantly disappears when the blower pump is turned off, the bed setting and supporting the patient. This makes moving and nursing procedures far easier than with the water bed. Also the upward draught of warm air ensures a healthy dry skin environment. Unfortunately the beds are bulky, heavy, and expensive (£57 a day hire charge). They are perhaps best reserved for special hospital departments such as intensive care units.

Mechanical beds

These reduce the duration of pressure on vulnerable sites by facilitating patient turning. The most common in general use is the net suspension bed. Other complex mechanical beds have been designed for use in special departments, such as spinal injury units where there is a need to turn patients who require absolute immobilisation. Electric turning beds are also available.

Net suspension beds consist of a slightly elastic open net mesh, wound round and suspended from two rollers. The net is lined by a blanket or sheet, which thus supports the patient by moulding to the body contours, so minimising point loading and also allowing skin ventilation. Patient turning is achieved by simply winding the net on to one roller by using an integral handle while unwinding the other. Although net beds have gained widespread use, there is little evidence for their effectiveness. They have been popular as labour saving nursing aids, but they may be less acceptable to patients who find themselves "on display" with restricted movement. They are easy to assemble and maintain, but it may be difficult to gauge the correct tension for the net: too low and the patient is unable to move, too high and tissue deformation occurs. Net beds may offer special advantages to patients who are at risk of pressure sores and who have painful conditions exacerbated by regular manual turning regimens, such as in generalised severe arthritis.

Selecting pressure relieving systems

The large range of pressure relieving systems and the complexity of some is daunting. A comprehensive list is provided by the Disabled Living Foundation. Few reports of comparative studies are available to guide selection and, disappointingly, most manufacturers provide only sparse objective supportive evidence for their product(s). The minimum information should include laboratory studies of pressure relieving characteristics and clinical trial data. Manufacturers should be more active in evaluating their products.

The Vaperm mattress is a well established prevention aid and should be considered for departments where vulnerable patients are often admitted, such as geriatric and orthopaedic wards. Large cell ripple mattresses are effective but continue to suffer from poor reliability. Padding overlays are also effective and easier to use in hospital or at home. The air wave system is valuable for those patients at high risk of pressure sores and is easier to use and considerably cheaper than air support systems. Both can be hired at daily rates rather than purchased.

The incidence of pressure sores is one of the few measures that indicate quality of care and should therefore be constantly monitored by all wards and departments. Aids are important in prevention but need to be readily available, clean, and well maintained. Ensuring education of staff about what to use, how to use it, and when is also important. These aspects of countering pressure sores cross health service departments and are therefore best addressed by a broad district wide approach. Each district should have a detailed pressure sore prevention policy with a stated means of implementation, monitoring and constant improvement. Unfortunately few health districts have awoken as yet to this simple but highly cost effective approach.

1 Scales JT, Lowthian PT, Poole AG, Ludman WR. "Vaperm" patient support system: a new general purpose hospital mattress. *Lancet* 1982;**ii**:1150–2.
2 Versluysen M. How elderly people with femoral fracture develop pressure sores in hospital. *Br Med J* 1986;**292**:1311–13.
3 Barratt E. A review of risk assessment methods. *Care, Science and Practice* 1988;**6**:49–52.
4 Exton-Smith AN, Sherwin RW. The prevention of pressure sores: significance of spontaneous bodily movements. *Lancet* 1961;**ii**:1124–6.
5 Barbenel JC, Jordan MM, Nicol SM, Clark MO. Incidence of pressure sores in the Greater Glasgow Health Board Area. *Lancet* 1977;**ii**:548–50.
6 Denne WA. An objective assessment of the sheepskins used for decubitus sore prophylaxis. *Rheumatology and Rehabilitation* 1979;**18**:23–9
7 Hughes AW. Prevention of pressure sores in patients with fractures of the femoral neck. *Injury* 1986;**17**:19–22.
8 Stapleton M. Preventing pressure sores—an evaluation of three products. *Geriatr Nurs (New York)* 1986 March/April:23–5.
9 Goldstone LA, Norris M, O'Reilly M, White J. A clinical trial of a bead system for the prevention of pressure sores in elderly orthopaedic patients. *J Adv Nurs* 1982;**7**:545–8
10 Bliss MR, McLaren R, Exton-Smith AN. Preventing pressure sores in hospital: controlled trial of a large celled ripple mattress. *Br Med J* 1967;**i**:394–7.
11 Bliss M. The use of ripple beds. *Age Ageing* 1978;**7**:25–7.
12 Exton Smith AN, Overstall PW, Wedgewood J, Wallace G. Use of the "air wave system" to prevent pressure sores in hospital. *Lancet* 1982;**i**:1288–90.
13 Redfern SJ, Jeneid PA, Gillingham ME, Lunn HF. Local pressures with ten types of patient support system. *Lancet* 1973;**ii**:277–80.

Appendix

Useful addresses

Society for Tissue Viability. Wessex Rehabilitation Association, Odstock Hospital, Salisbury, Wiltshire SP2 8BJ.

King's Fund Pressure Sore Group. Professor B Liversley, Department of the Care of the Elderly, St Stephen's Hospital, Fulham Road, London SW10 0TH.

Disabled Living Foundation. Disability Equipment Handbook, Pressure Relief (Section 1B), 380/384 Harrow Road, London W9 2HU (071 289 6111). The Disabled Living Foundation will provide the address of your local Disabled Living Centre, which provides helpful advice on equipment for disability.

Bed aids for home nursing

AF TRAVERS, PW BELFIELD

The able bodied among us spend a third of our lives in bed. We take for granted our ability to turn over and get up when we please. In contrast, the disabled patient may spend considerably longer in bed and may have difficulty moving in the bed or getting in and out of it. Many aids and accessories are available and these fall into two broad categories: those for improving mobility around the bed and those for comfort.

Mobility aids

These aim at improving independence in movement on the bed and help in getting in and out of the bed. The type of bed—for example, a simple divan or a loaned hospital bed—will influence fixation of the aid to the bed. Most aids therefore come in several forms, depending on which bed is used.

Lifting (monkey) poles (fig 1) consist of a cantilever gantry with a support chain or strap from which hangs a handle. They are used to help the patient raise himself or herself off the bed or to move up the bed and their usefulness depends on good strength in the arms. They are most useful for paraplegic patients and other people with problems with their legs. The handle should be large enough for two hands, and the support strap should be adjusted to the correct length, just near enough for the patient to grasp the handle from a lying position. Attendants should take care to avoid head injury on the dangling handle. The lifting pole must be well anchored—that is, clamped to a hospital type bed or screwed to a divan—and its stability should be checked in use. Direct fixing to the ceiling or wall is also possible. Costs range from £40 to £150.

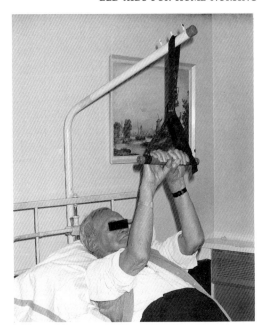

FIG 1—Lifting pole

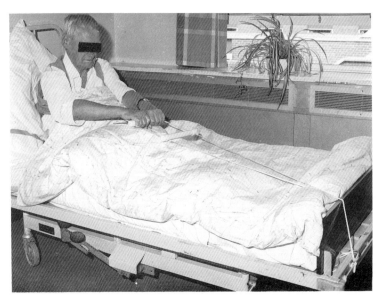

FIG 2—Rope ladder

Rope ladders (fig 2) enable the user to pull himself or herself up from lying to a sitting position and require strength in both arms as the user "climbs" the ladder, rung by rung. They are fixed to the foot of the bed and usually consist of synthetic ropes with wooden or plastic rungs. They are cheap at £5 to £10.

Grab handles (fig 3) help patients to get into and out of bed and are particularly useful for those with unilateral hemiparesis. They also provide something to pull on for movements around the bed. They are adjustable in height and rotate through 360°, locking in eight different positions (for example, the Divan Bed Aid). The most commonly used types are the Lewisham and King's Fund frames, which clamp on to hospital type beds, and the Divan Bed Aid, which screws to the floor and the bed. Firm anchorage is important: patients and their carers should be shown by a nurse or therapist how to use the grab handle. Costs vary from £45 to £60.

A Manchester bed raise bar helps people to get in and out of bed. It is a horizontal bar screwed to the frame of the bed so that the bar runs level with the top of the mattress. The user can pull on the bar. She or he can also use it for counter pressure when attempting to rise from sitting on the side of the bed, when the bar provides firmer support than a sprung mattress. The cost is about £22.

Cot sides and side rails—There is a wide range of these available and many are adjustable for height and width (fig 4). They can be fitted to domestic divans. When not in use they fold or drop down. They provide a rail for patients to pull on to enable turning over in bed. They can prevent rolling out of bed, but they should not be used as a method of restraint as determined and restless patients will climb over them (and thus fall from an even greater height) and may injure their legs.[1] For these reasons their routine use should be avoided. Costs range from £40 to £120.

Bed raisers—It is difficult to stand from sitting on a low bed. People with muscle wasting or joint stiffness find getting up easier from a higher bed. Wheelchair users need a bed of the same height as the wheelchair, usually about 48 cm, or higher if a wheelchair cushion is used. The commonest type of bed raiser is the wooden block, which can increase the height of the bed off the floor by 7 to 25 cm (fig 5). Screw in extensions for divan bed legs are also available. Other reasons for selectively raising the head or the foot of the bed respectively are reflux oesophagitis and ankle swelling. A set of bed blocks costs under £10.

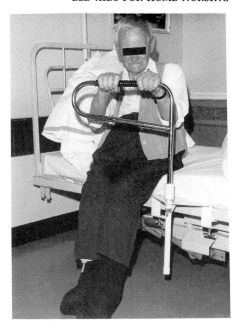

FIG 3—Grab handle

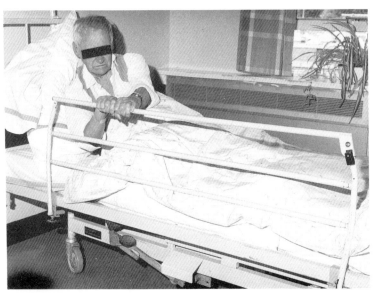

FIG 4—Side rail

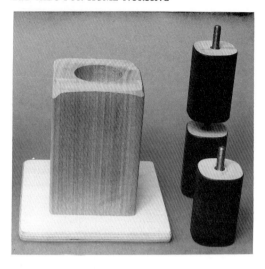

FIG 5—Bed raisers

Aids for comfort

Backrests adjust to different positions and fold flat when not in use. The frames are metal or wooden. Pneumatic mattress raisers can be placed between the bed base and the mattress and a handheld control system allows the patient to lower or raise the bedhead into variable positions. A backrest costs between £10 and £40.

Wedges and support pillows—Like backrests these provide comfort and support, enabling the user to sit up in bed, but may lead to the user sliding forward as the flexed position of the hips is unopposed by any flexion of the knees. This can be prevented by raising the foot of the bed a few centimetres. In patients with problems with sensation or severe weakness of the legs, however, this measure will not prevent the increased risk of pressure sores caused by the forward slide. Pillows should be flame retardant and washable. The "wishbone" shaped pillow supports the back, shoulders, arms, and neck. A wide range of foam wedge supports is available for use under legs, shoulders, and back, and to help positioning in bed. The costs range from £10 to £50.

Bed cradles (fig 6) support the weight of bedclothes over a patient's legs and feet. They are cantilever in shape and are usually made of coated tubular steel. They are anchored by sliding under the mattress. Some fold when not in use for easier storage.

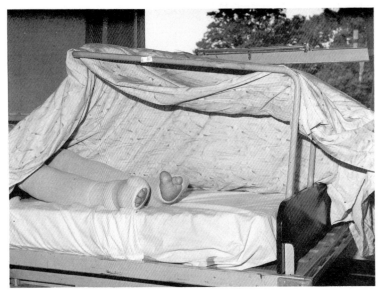

FIG 6—Bed cradle

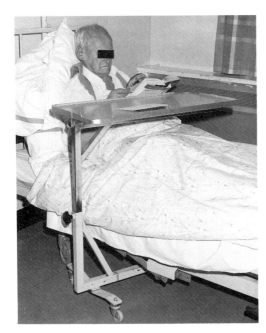

FIG 7—Cantilever bed
table

Disadvantages of their use are the possible risk of trauma to the legs and that they may make the legs or feet cold. They cost £10 to £25.

Bed mirrors—Viewing mirrors clamped to the side of the bed may enable the user to see more of her or his environment.

Bed tables—There are over 70 types of bed table available. The commonest is the cantilever table (fig 7). These may have press button height and tilt adjustment to suit individual needs. Usually the base has castors to allow movement and open ended legs to slip easily under the bed. Most tables have lipped edges to prevent objects rolling off the top. Some tables are overbed—that is, bridge shaped—and others are trays on folding legs. Book rests and reading frames, some with devices for turning pages, are also available.

Provision of aids and accessories

There are no formal studies of the provision, use, and usefulness of the equipment discussed above nor of the number of people at home who have difficulty with mobility in bed and with transfers into and out of bed. We know from clinical experience that people with stroke and Parkinson's disease often have such problems.

Bed aids needed for home nursing are usually supplied free of charge by health authorities. Social services may supply some of the aids designed for comfort, but there is widespread variation in arrangements.[2] Unfortunately, the vast range of bed aids makes it possible for people (or families acting on their behalf) to buy or accept aids that are not fully appropriate for their needs. Proper assessment including home visits by the occupational therapist and nursing staff will avoid these problems.[3] Further information can be obtained from books and leaflets,[4] and if possible a visit to a disabled living centre should be made.[5] Doctors and other health workers can make use of the numerous aids and accessories that are available to improve appreciably the quality of home life for the patient "stranded" in bed.

1 Coakley D. On the dangers of getting out of bed in hospital. *Health Trends* 1980;**12**:5–6.
2 Mulley GP. Provision of aids. *Br Med J* 1988;**296**:1317–18.
3 Jay P. *Coping with disability*. London: Disabled Living Foundation, 1984.
4 Disabled Living Foundation. Beds and bed accessories. In: *Disabled Living Foundation Information Handbook*. London: Disabled Living Foundation, 1989. (Section 1A, ISD No 83/2.)
5 Chamberlain MA. Disabled living centres. *Br Med J* 1988;**296**:1052–3.

Dressing aids

SCM MITCHELL

Dressing difficulties are widespread—for example, half of rheumatology outpatients have some difficulty.[1] A survey of people aged over 75 and living at home found that over 92% were independent in dressing, with about 5·5% needing help and 1·5% using an aid.[2] Only half of those in residential homes and 16% of those in nursing homes, however, were able to dress or wash without help.[3] Most surveys have found general ignorance about dressing aids and in particular where to obtain them.[1 2 4] Devices that help in dressing should not substitute for advice on appropriate clothing, its adaptation and material, or the development of dressing techniques specific to a person's needs. Many patients can be helped by being shown different methods of dressing. Thus, prior assessment by an occupational therapist may best direct the provision of aids. The key criteria for a successful dressing aid are that it should be easy to use, light, and resilient.

Reaching aids—Pick up or reaching aids benefit patients with restricted reach or difficulties with balance and range from lightweight to heavy duty. The basic features are gripping jaws, which may incorporate a magnet, a metal stem ranging from 40 to 125 cm in length, and a hand grip with trigger to open and close the jaws (fig 1). Prices range from £5 to over £65 depending on materials and attachments. When choosing a reaching aid it is important to consider the weight, hand grip, length, and main area of use of the aid. Reasonable coordination is required, particularly for the folding lazy tong type. A 60 cm length may be appropriate for use while sitting but over 80 cm will be needed while standing. Too long an aid, however, will hinder retrieval where there is limited shoulder movement.[5] Folding reachers or ones that clip on to a frame or stick enable the aid to be carried, extending its area of use. Patients with weak arms or hands will require a lightweight aid,

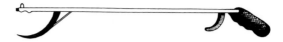

FIG 1—Reaching aid

perhaps with a broad trigger and locking action to reduce the need for a sustained grip. Arm supports or a two handed grip can be incorporated to help those with weak wrists. The range of objects to be picked up will dictate the strength and size of jaw opening required and whether rotation of the jaws is needed.

Dressing sticks are commercially available but can be simply made by adapting a wooden coathanger (fig 2). The central hook is removed and a cuphook screwed into one end of the hanger. A rubber thimble, to which clothing will cling, can be placed on the other end or a notch cut into the wood. The aid can then be used to lift clothes or straps up over the shoulder when there is limited shoulder movement or weak arms. The hook can be used to pull up zips after attaching a keyring to the zip or catch loops sewn into garments. When there are difficulties bending, clothes can be pushed down by the notched or thimbled ends. The stick will substitute for a reaching aid when there is poor manual dexterity or insufficient finger strength. A piece of webbing tacked on to the hanger allows the aid to be used when there is inadequate grip. For many the standard walking stick may double as dressing stick.

Button hooks consist of a wooden handle and wire loop and enable buttons to be fastened with one hand. The button is captured within the loop, which has already passed through the button hole, and the button and loop are pulled back through the hole. By twisting the button hook the button is released, but good vision and function of the hands are needed. A more recent alternative is the one handed toggle button hook (fig 3). Pressing the plastic handles opens out the loop enabling the button to be caught. The button is pulled through the hole and released by

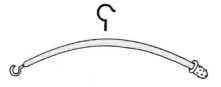

FIG 2—Dressing stick

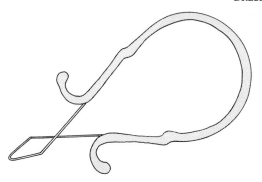

FIG 3—Toggle button aid

further pressure on the plastic handles. The aid is light and easier to use than the original button hook.

Stocking and sock aids—There are many varieties of stocking aid, though most are unpopular, subjects finding the aid requires more effort than no aid.[6] Up to 45% of a mixed group of patients did not use their prescribed stocking aids, this being particularly common in the 70–80 age group.[7] Stocking aids are useful where there is limited hip movement or restricted bending—for example, in the early days after hip replacement—but most require reasonable manual dexterity to place the stocking on to the aid or even to assemble it. Stocking aids usually take the form of a gutter or rigid structure over which the stocking is stretched, the aid is lowered to the floor and the foot placed inside the gutter, the combined stocking and gutter being pulled up the leg by means of tapes or handles. A survey into eight types of stocking aid came out strongly in favour of the travel sock aid.[7] This consists of an outer cloth cover over an inner plastic shape (fig 4). The stocking grips to the cloth and the aid is pulled up the leg by means of tapes. Hand grip can be improved by tying knots into the tapes. This is no longer available but the similar flexible sock and stocking aid (Nottingham Rehab and Helping Hand Company) comprising a low friction inner nylon surface and outer terry towelling cover with looped tapes (fig 5) is effective. Other recommended aids were the Swedish one handed sock aid (Llewellyn Health Care Services) (fig 6) and the Dorking stocking gutter (fig 7).[7] The stocking gutter is greatly improved from the standard gutter type by its shorter gutter and deeper notches, which better retain the stocking.

31

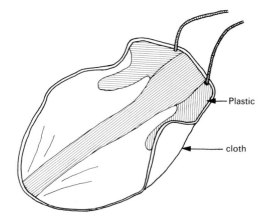

FIG 4—Travel sock aid

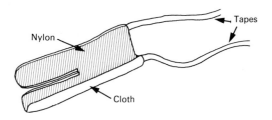

FIG 5—Flexible sock and stocking aid

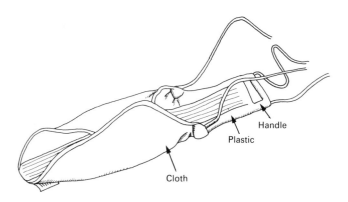

FIG 6—One handed sock aid

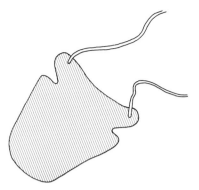

FIG 7—Dorking stocking gutter

Similar types of aid are made by several companies. The cloth type aids are efficient and comfortable and suit most weights of sock or stocking but are more expensive than the plastic gutter types. The fabric dress aid consists of two long fabric tongues that are fixed together and fed into the stocking, which is attached to the aid by suspenders. It is rather cumbersome but comfortable. Tight aids are usually in the form of conjointed stocking aids. The Swedish version consists of two one handed stocking aids held together by a clip, the clip falling off at midcalf. The double stocking gutter requires excellent hand function to feed the tights on to the aid. Both types of aid take the tights to the knee with the remaining difficulty of pulling the tights over the hips when there is poor hand or shoulder function. Thus, though useful for patients with limited hip movement, they may not be appropriate for those disabled with rheumatoid arthritis or stroke. There is no suitable appliance for putting on elastic stockings. Both the elastic stocking aid frame and the elastic stocking aid gutter have been found to be extremely difficult to use by both patients and controls, a particular problem being feeding the stocking on to the aid.

Shoe horns are commonly used by elderly patients, being used by a fifth of subjects in one survey of patients aged over 80.[8] Factors to consider when choosing a shoe horn are the mode of putting on shoes and the degree of spinal rotation and ankle movement. For those who can stand or who have poor hip movement a long shoe horn is preferable, the optimum length being between 53 and 62 cm.[7] When there is limited back mobility or reduced ankle movement a shoe horn with a stiff spring will help. The length of leg from knee to heel should be assessed, too long a shoe horn being difficult to use from a sitting position. Shoe horns with a built up handle are available to improve grip. The most popular plastic shoe horn has a hook handle that can help pull on other items of clothing but is only 43 cm long.

Shoe levers usually take the form of a large notch cut into a plastic or wood frame and help removal of shoes or boots. The aid is stabilised with one foot and the other shoe placed into the cutout shape, eliminating the need to bend. Evaluation of boot removers showed the Bootsoff version to be more efficient than the wooden shoe remover (Homecraft), which is unstable on carpeted floors.[7] Alternatively, a notched dressing stick may be adequate, provided the edges do not catch the skin or stockings. In practice, however, it is usually safer to sit down and lever the shoe off with the other foot.

Shoe ties help patients who can bend but have poor manual dexterity or loss of function in one hand, eliminating the need to tie shoe laces. The No Bows aid is a spring loaded shoe lace aid. The laces are threaded through the aid, knotted to form a loop, and gripped by the spring. Pressing the two ends of the aid together releases the laces, which are tightened by sliding the aid up the laces while tethering the looped end with the little finger (fig 8). Although marketed for one handed use, two hands are required to assemble the aid and a strong pinch grip is required between thumb and forefinger with good finger coordination. Evaluation in patients with rheumatoid arthritis showed only 14% were able to press the spring together.[1] They may be of help, however, to patients with a stroke. Alternatively laces can be fastened by Velcro

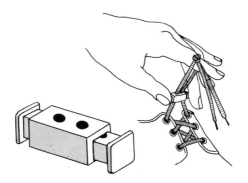

FIG 8—Spring loaded lace aid

by using a hooked dressing stick (fig 9). Details on one handed tying methods can be obtained from the Disabled Living Foundation. Fastening the shoe with wide Velcro straps will eliminate the need for laces.

Elastic shoe laces enable laceup shoes to be slipped on with the help of a shoe horn without untying the laces and are thus helpful for those with restricted hip flexion or poor hand function. Shoes tied with elastic laces, however, provide less support than ordinary laces. To avoid the tongue of the shoe being trapped when the shoe is put on either the laces can be inserted through the tongue or a hole made into it through which the hook of a dressing aid can be inserted. Elastic laces come in three sizes from most major suppliers and have an approximate life span of three months.

Fasteners—Onehanded fasteners appropriate for weak or one-handed use include Kempner and Velcro types. The Kempner fastener consists of a sliding hook and bar threaded on to tape or webbing (fig 10). Garments can be closed without tension by attaching the hook to the bar and then tightened by pulling on the tape. Pulling in the opposite direction loosens the tape. Edgeware

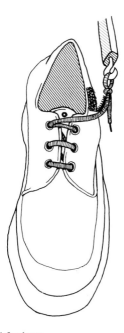

FIG 9—Hooked dressing aid for laces

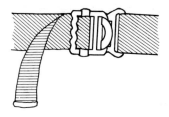

FIG 10—Kempner fastener

braces are elastic braces with a single point of attachment at the back and are worn like a school satchel (fig 11). Trousers can be lowered without removing overgarments by releasing a Velcro fastening on either side at the front of the braces, allowing braces to be extended. The pattern is obtained from the clothing advisory service of the Disabled Living Foundation.

The zippade is a long cord with a hook that fits into the pull of the zip helping those with limited dexterity. It is available in haberdashery shops.

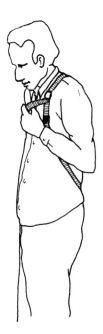

FIG 11—Edgeware brace

Clip on ties can be attached one handed over the top button of the shirt collar and may be useful to hemiplegic or parkinsonian patients.

Where to obtain aids

Wherever possible aids should be tried before purchase. The disabled living centres will demonstrate and advise on a wide range of aids but do not sell any appliances. Occupational therapists are available to patients in hospital and at home through the social services. Although some local authorities will lend out aids on a long term basis, others require the aid to be purchased. Ideally, aids should be available on loan, perhaps for a trial period, before purchase. Although aids are available through mail order catalogues, prior assessment through either disabled living centre or occupational therapists is advised.

I thank Linda Tomlinson, senior occupational therapist, Bradford Royal Infirmary, for her help in preparing the manuscript.

1 Howell C. Survey into the prevalence of dressing problems. In: *An assessment of the use of lower limb dressing aids*. Publications Unit, No 2 Site, Manchester Road, Heywood, Lancashire, Department of Health and Social Security, 1986.
2 Clarke M, Clarke S, Odell A, Jagger C. The elderly at home: health and social status. *Health Trends* 1984;**16**:3–7.
3 Clarke M, Hughes AO, Dodd KJ, *et al*. The elderly in residential care: patterns of disability. *Health Trends* 1979;**11**:17–20.
4 Chamberlain MA, Stowe J. A survey of personal aids supplied by post to arthritics. *Rheumatology and Rehabilitation*. 1980;**19**:246–51.
5 Dawkins ME. *Report of an assessment of long handed reachers at Middlesbrough general hospital*. Lancashire: Department of Health and Social Security, 1986.
6 Howell C. Survey into the usage of stocking aids. In: *An assessment of the use of lower limb dressing aids*. Lancashire: Department of Health and Social Security, 1986.
7 Howell C. *An assessment of the use of lower limb dressing aids*. Lancashire: Department of Health and Social Security, 1986.
8 White E, Mulley GP. Footwear worn by the over 80's: a community survey. *Clinical Rehabilitation* 1989;**3**:23–5.

Appendix

Useful addresses/publications

Disabled Living Foundation Clothing Advisor, 380–384 Harrow Road, London W9 2HU (071 289 6111). Advice by post (send sae) or visit by appointment. The Disabled Living Foundation produces a series of books on clothing needs and dressing for the disabled, details of which can be obtained from Haigh and

Hochland, The Precinct Centre, Oxford Road, Manchester M13 9QA (061 273 4156). The Disabled Living Foundation will provide the address of your local Disabled Living Centre, which provides helpful advice on equipment for disability.

Clothing and dressing for the disabled. In: *Disabled Living Foundation Service Handbook*. 5th ed 1981. Oxford: Equipment for the Disabled, Mary Marlborough Lodge, 1981.

Fashion Services for the Disabled, Units B270–B320, Saltaire Workshops, Ashley Lane, Shipley, West Yorkshire BD17 7SR (0274 597487). Training and research centre into clothing needs. Free courses. Workshop designs and makes garments to meet individual needs.

The Scottish Council on Disability, Princes House, 5 Shandwick Place, Edinburgh EH2 4RG.

Turnbull P, Ruston R. *Clothes Sense for Disabled People of all Ages*. Purley: Piel Caru, 1985.

Jay P. *Coping with Disability*. London: Disabled Living Foundation, 1984.

Darnborough A, Kinrade D. *Directory of Aids for Disabled and Elderly People*. Cambridge: Woodhead-Faulkner, 1986.

Manufacturers

Notingham Rehab, Customer Service Department, 17 Ludlow Hill Road, West Bridgeford, Nottingham NG2 6HD (0602 234251). Mail order catalogue *Ways and Means* from Freepost, Nottingham NG2 1BR.

Boots the Chemists, Medical Merchandise Department, Nottingham NG2 3AA. Booklet *Healthcare in the Home* from any Boots store. Home delivery service.

Homecraft Supplies Ltd, 27 Trinity Road, London SW17 7SF (081 672 7070)

The Helping Hand Company, Mecanaids Ltd, St Catherine Street, Gloucester GL1 2SL (0452 500200).

RSFU Sweden. Aids obtainable through Llewellyn Health Care Services, Carlton Street, Liverpool L3 7ED (051 236 5311).

British Red Cross, Medical Aids Department, 76 Clarendon Park Road, Leicester LE2 3AD.

Emergency alarms

KEREN N DAVIES

Emergency alarms can extend the care provided to disabled and vulnerable elderly people who may be unsupervised at home for much of the day and all night. The availability of alarms has widened because of the increasing number of people over 75 and a trend towards care of disabled people in the community.

Alarms are advocated for people at risk. Risk is loosely defined and might include the physically impaired, the socially isolated (living alone or with someone unable to help in an emergency), those who tend to fall, perhaps those living in poorer housing, and the very old. Any person able to operate the alarm and understand its purpose may be eligible.

Types of alarms

Simple alarms

Simple indicators such as cards to place in a window, systems of lights, bells, or buzzers, and even whistles have been tried without success. Except for whistles (if carried) all need to be activated from a single point or require the person in need to remain mobile and dextrous. The response depends on willing neighbours and relatives, who carry a heavy burden of responsibility. Twenty four hour cover can rarely be given, and the person's vulnerability is advertised.

Telephones can be used in an emergency to summon help, but 6% of people over 75 and 20% of those over 85 have difficulties using them.[1] In a situation of stress these proportions are even higher: in 46% of accidents the victim cannot reach the telephone or dial.[2]

Emergency alarms

Dispersed alarms are single unit alarms that enable residents in individual dwellings to make emergency calls. Radiotransmission or telephone based systems automatically dial either a single contact point or a sequence of prearranged numbers of relatives and friends. When several elderly people live in a small geographical area their alarms can be wired to a central (unstaffed) unit, often at a warden's flat. The signals can then be relayed by radio or telephone to the emergency centre. These grouped systems can be cheaper than true dispersed alarms.

Emergency centres are staffed for 24 hours every day. The operators have access to a computer database with details of the resident and nominated respondents. They respond to the call by telephoning wardens, relatives, home care teams, volunteers, or the emergency services and asking them to visit the resident.

There are several makes of emergency alarm, but most comprise a home alarm unit, a triggering device, and a link to an emergency centre. Figure 1 shows an example of an alarm unit, comprising combined telephone and alarm unit activated by pressing the red button on the unit or portable trigger, which may be worn as a clothes clip (fig 2) or a pendant. The home unit may not include a telephone, and in sheltered accommodation the units are usually only alarms and wall mounted, requiring a power supply. The alarm is activated by a button or pull cord on the unit.

Alternative triggers may be portable radio devices (pendant, clothes clip, or wrist strap) that activate the unit from a variable distance (most will work from any point in a three bedroomed house and usually in the immediate grounds) or fixed triggers—for example, ceiling mounted pull cords or wall mounted push buttons. Fixed triggers are less satisfactory as they are usually too far above the ground to be reached after a fall. Once triggered the alarm unit will put out a call. The unit may be preset to dial a sequence of friends' or relatives' telephone numbers and then play a prerecorded message to summon help or put a call through to the emergency centre (fig 3).

Innovations

There have been several new developments in alarm systems since their introduction. Fifteen out of 20 alarms on the market have a built in loudspeaker and microphone that allows two way

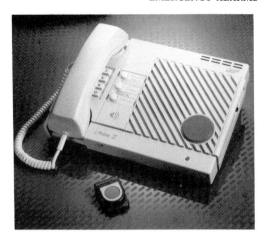

FIG 1—Piper Lifeline II and trigger

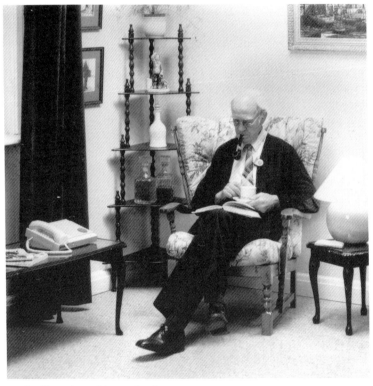

FIG 2—Alarm in position on lapel

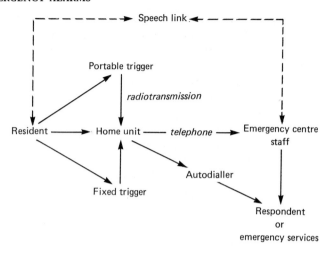

FIG 3—Call sequence for emergency alarm

speech between the resident and emergency centre even if the resident cannot reach the home unit. Alternative triggers may be installed to activate the alarm—for example, smoke detectors and intruder alarms. An "inactivity" feature may be included in the home unit. These units have a 12 or 24 hour timer that is reset each time the unit is used. If unused or not reset in a predetermined period a call is automatically sent out. Some new alarms work on a "habit cycle system" and send out an alarm call if a specific event, such as water being drawn from the water main, does not take place within a predetermined period. An interface such as the Wolsey cat has been developed, which creates compatibility between different manufacturers' alarms and control centre computers.

Problems with alarms

One in six residents sustaining an accident or fall cannot activate an alarm.[3] Even if a habit cycle is included the waiting period for help may be eight to 24 hours. Alarms are underused and most often used in non-critical situations. In one study 81% of 608 residents in sheltered housing had not used their alarms in an emergency over one year and 7% had not been able to activate the alarm in an emergency.[4] In another survey over half of residents had used the alarm at some time but only one third had done so in an emergency.[2] Most alarm systems are linked to sheltered housing, and the supply of housing can no longer meet the increased demand. Therefore many people at risk are not covered by the present systems.

Systems using radio transmission used to suffer from problems of interference from continental broadcasting stations and local authority systems that used similar equipment. To rectify this the Department of Trade and Industry designated specific frequencies for use by local authority alarm systems. Licences for operating a radio alarm are given only to local authorities. The emergency centres have to be in the locality of the population using the radio alarm, whereas telephone based systems can be linked to emergency centres anywhere in the country. The cost of radio alarms is variable because of the need for an external aerial mast.

Demand for alarms has not come from residents, and alarm installation has escalated without any formal evidence of need or demand for the system being collected. Alarms do, however, give reassurance to both the residents and their relatives. The alarms do not result in reduced contact between the housebound and their families or the professional services.[2] The use of alarms depends on the attitude of the users and, when living in sheltered housing, the relationship with their warden; over half of interviewed residents said they would not like to live without their alarms.[2]

Referrals are considered from all health and social workers but may be accepted from relatives when supported by a medical opinion. Even if a resident is not eligible for a local authority alarm he or she may still be able to link into a local authority emergency centre with an alarm bought privately (so long as it is compatible with the local authority system). Sixty local authorities offer a monitoring service to residents anywhere in the United Kingdom but because of variations in determining who responds to the call it is usually better to use the nearest centre.

Provision of alarms

Some manufacturers sell or rent alarms direct to the public. Some companies run their own emergency monitoring centres. Those who do not will be able to advise on the nearest suitable centre. The Disabled Living Foundation provides information on alarm systems, which is available to the public.

Help the Aged offers advice on alarms and has a scheme to

provide alarms and organise monitoring for people in most parts of the United Kingdom. There is often a waiting list for an alarm, and if means allow a donation of £220 is expected. When the alarm is no longer required it should be returned. Three charities have an established service to sell or rent units and arrange monitoring. Care Trust sells alarm units and offers monitoring anywhere in the United Kingdom. It provides an emergency centre for the London Borough of Tower Hamlets. The Home Call Trust rents units and offers monitoring at £12 a month if residents can afford it. The trust covers south west England. Oxfordshire Council for Voluntary Service sells or rents units to residents in Oxfordshire and calls are monitored by Oxfordshire central ambulance control. Other charities, such as the British Legion, may be able to help with the costs of alarms provided to war pensioners.

Many private housing associations include alarm systems in their developments, which link into local emergency centres. They can be found under housing associations, societies, and trusts in the Yellow Pages telephone directory. The commonest way to obtain an alarm, however, is from the local housing or social services department. Authorities vary as to who controls the allocation and provision of alarms. The address and telephone number of the relevant department can be found in the telephone directory. There are currently more than 300 schemes that operate either by radiotransmission or telephone. Many are an integral part of sheltered housing complexes or linked to warden supervision; some authorities provide alarms to other residents. Many authorities run their own emergency centres, and others use commercial centres. The cost of provision, maintenance, and monitoring varies throughout the country. Although the service may be provided free to residents, some authorities make a charge and use this revenue to help finance the service. Most funding comes from a single departmental budget, but in some areas there are contributions from the area health authority and housing departments. Specific details should be sought from the local departments.

Costs of alarms

Alarms may be expensive for many old people but relatives sometimes buy them as Christmas or birthday presents. If residents are buying or renting alarms they must decide if they require a monitoring service. The cheapest option is a preset autodialling unit. If monitoring is required then the unit should be compatible with the emergency centre with the lowest monitoring costs and free monitoring space.

The items for costing include the cost of installing a telephone line, converting the socket, and renting the line; the cost of renting an alarm and monitoring (local authorities may not charge but usually the charge ranges from £80 to £160 a year; commercial firms charge about £250 for the first year and £150 for subsequent years); and the cost of buying an alarm, which ranges from £170 to £320, and monitoring fees (local authorities or charities charge £10 to £70 a year and commercial firms charge £20 to £150 a year). Alarms are zero rated for value added tax if supplied to someone who is chronically sick or disabled. Details are obtainable from the local taxation office.

I thank Tunstall Telecom, Whiteley Lodge, Whiteley Bridge, Yorkshire, for providing the photographs.

1 Hunt A. *The elderly at home.* London: Office of Population Censuses and Surveys. HMSO, 1978.
2 Research Institute for Consumer Affairs. *Dispersed alarm systems: a guide for organisations installing systems.* London: Research Institute for Consumer Affairs (RICA), 1986.
3 Feeney R, Galer M, Gallagher M. *Alarm systems for elderly and disabled people.* Loughborough Institute of Consumer Ergonomics, 1981.
4 Wilcocks AJ. *Care and housing of the elderly in the community.* Nottingham: Institute of Social Welfare, 1979.

Appendix

Useful addresses

Help the Aged, Community Alarms Department, 16–18 St James's Walk, London (071 253 0253).
Research Unit for Consumer Affairs, 2 Marylebone Road, London NW1 4DX. An information pack, *Alarms for Elderly People,* is available from this address.
Wolsey Electronics Ltd, Gellihirion Industrial Estate, Pontypridd, Mid Glamorgan CF37 5SX (044385 3111).
Disabled Living Foundation, 380–384 Harrow Road, London W9 2HU (071 289 6111). The Disabled Living Foundation will provide the address of your local Disabled Living Centre, which provides helpful advice on equipment for disability.
Care Trust, Care House, Bigland Street, London E1 2ND.
The Home Call Trust, 34 Logan Road, Bristol BS7 8DR.
Oxfordshire Council for Voluntary Service, Pratten Building, New Road, Oxford OX1 1ND.

Feeding aids

M J CONNOLLY, A S WILSON

Although problems with eating and drinking are not confined to elderly people, 3% of those over 65 living at home have difficulties and 2–4% of those over 85 cannot feed independently.[1] Independent feeding or drinking, or both, may prove difficult for many reasons (box).

Common causes of feeding difficulties in adults

Impairment	Examples of cause
Impaired body posture	Tetraplegia, hemiplegia
Lost use of one arm	Hemiplegia, amputation
Impairment of use of both arms (due to pain, weakness, sensory changes, stiffness, tremor)	Tetraplegia, bilateral stroke, rheumatoid arthritis, neuropathies, parkinsonism
Swallowing difficulties	Facial, bulbar, and pseudobulbar palsy
Cognitive impairment	Alzheimer's disease, cerebrovascular dementia

---

Some general points are worthy of emphasis. Firstly, disabled people often eat slowly; food must be hot to begin with to remain appetising. Secondly, a table and chair of correct height are vital for maximum comfort and efficiency[2 3]; and thirdly, the type of food is as important as the utensils—for example, soups are difficult for those with tremor and hand held foods such as sandwiches are easy for hemiplegics or blind people.[3]

Of all aids for disabled people feeding aids are among those prescribed least often[4] and perhaps least often used.[5] Aids may maintain independence and dignity,[6] but patients often develop other ways of coping and aids are not always beneficial, especially if patients regard them as unattractive ("ugly mugs") or as drawing attention to their disability. Furthermore, patients often buy (perhaps expensive) aids commercially to find them of little benefit.[3] Before aids are tried it is wise to confirm that the patient's inability to manage conventional equipment is caused by his or her disability and not by defective conventional utensils (Is the knife sharp enough?). Three basic guidelines for providing feeding (or any) aids are, firstly, obtain professional assessment from an occupational therapist; secondly, provide aids only when other ways of coping fail; and, thirdly, supply aids that are simple and look as normal and attractive as possible.

Feeding aids for specific disabilities

Loss of use of one arm

The main feeding difficulties for people who have lost an arm are maintaining a stable base (plate or dish), cutting up food, and getting food off the plate. Non-slip mats anchor the plate or cup to the table or tray. Only about a third of non-slip mats used in hospital stroke rehabilitation, however, are taken home on discharge.[5] Plates with basal suction pads serve the same purpose. Suction egg cups anchor to both table and egg (fig 1), and rocker

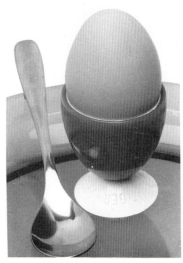

FIG 1—Suction egg cup

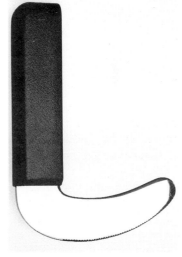

FIG 2—Amefa rocking knife

47

knives eliminate the need to stabilise food with the other hand (fig 2). Several varieties of combination knife and fork (with or without spoon) are marketed, but if these are deemed appropriate care is needed to choose one in which the cutting edge is not put in the mouth. Some of these devices can cut the angle of the mouth when used as a fork or spoon. In practice, however, many hemiplegic patients abandon trying to cut up food, choosing instead food that requires minimal or no cutting, or leave the task of cutting up food to the carer. To minimise "pea chasing," plastic plate guards, which clip to the plate rim, are useful, though unsightly. An increasing variety of attractive, deep, steep sided plates serve the same purpose (fig 3).[3]

Impaired use of both arms

Poor grip due to weakness, pain, or stiffness is helped by lightweight utensils with large handles.[2] Lightweight insulated mugs prevent burns to the hands in patients with sensory impairment or in those with weak grip who tend to steady the cup with the knuckles when gripping the handle. Mugs with two handles also help poor grip (fig 4)[3] as does the Manoy beaker, which is held between the thumb and index finger (fig 5), thus obviating the need for thumb opposition. The Doidy cup (fig 5) has an angled base

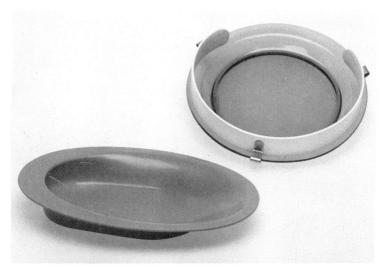

FIG 3—Steep sided plate (*left*) and plastic plate guard (*right*)

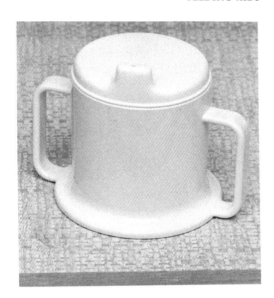

FIG 4—Two handled
spouted feeding cup

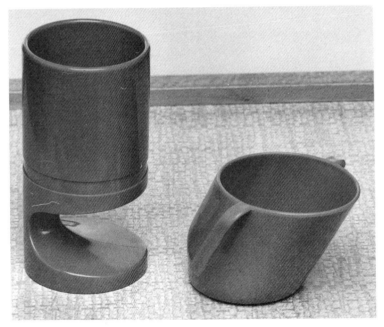

FIG 5—Manoy beaker (*left*) and Doidy cup (*right*)

and lip to help those who have difficulty with pronation (such as in parkinsonism). Unfortunately, many lightweight mugs are both unattractive and uninsulated.

Cutlery with large diameter lightweight handles is provided by several manufacturers (fig 6). A cheaper, though unattractive, alternative is to attach lightweight foam rubber plastazoate tubing (various diameters are available commercially) over the handles of conventional cutlery. When finger flexion is particularly weak but elbow movement is retained leather handstraps may be used to hold cutlery. A versatile alternative (Sunflower Selectagrip) provides multiple shapes and diameters of detachable handles that clip to a plastic handstrap. Some users, however, find the strap difficult to adjust.[2] Severe tremor, especially on intention, is particularly frustrating. Weighted wrist straps are said to minimise tremor, but we do not find these helpful and know of no objective evidence of their value. Capped cups, commonly with spouts, eliminate spillage, but patients are often embarrassed by what they perceive as baby cups (see fig 4). A simple alternative is to only half fill a large conventional mug. Cups with concave anti-splash lids (with holes not spouts) or flexible plastic "bendistraws" may also be more acceptable.

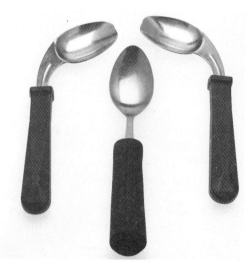

FIG 6—Angled spoons with large diameter handles on either side of ordinary spoon with foam rubber handle. Angled spoons require less wrist movement and are easier to place in mouth

Unilateral facial palsy

Unless mild, unilateral facial palsy causes dribbling of liquids and pouching of solids in the paralysed cheek (potentially dangerous as food may be aspirated when the patient is asleep). Cups with spouts (capped or not) may prevent dribbling. Conventional straws are less appropriate as the patient's ability to suck is usually impaired, but straws with a non-return valve (Pat Saunders straw) often solve the problem. Pouching is controlled simply by awareness of the phenomenon and inspection of the cheek pouch after meals and at bedtime.

Visual impairment

Large utensils of contrasting colours are sometimes valuable for people with visual impairment. Sectored plates are usually unnecessary,[3] provided food is arranged in a preset pattern. Deep plates or plate guards may, however, prevent food spillage, an otherwise common problem.[3]

Cognitive impairment

Independent feeding is sometimes impossible in demented subjects. More commonly feeding is either messy as use of more complicated equipment (such as knife fork coordination) proves difficult. The carer's frustration can be lessened simply by serving food that may be eaten with a spoon. Much of the equipment already discussed may also be helpful, but complex aids should be avoided. Cognitive impairment may reduce coordination of pronation as utensils are brought to the mouth. Indeed carers often say "She uses a spoon like a baby." This may be helped by the use of angled utensils (particularly spoons), which are available for right and left handed use (see fig 6).

Conclusion

The above guidelines are neither exhaustive nor universally applicable. Conversely, some aids described for one disability may be helpful for those with different problems (such as angled utensils for patients with parkinsonism). Advice on specific feeding problems can be provided by hospital and community based occupational therapists and by disabled living centres. Feeding aids should be attractive and normal to appeal to patients. Some

51

manufacturers have recently recognised this, and perhaps newer and better designed feeding aids will enjoy wider use. Although many feeding aids are available, there has been little objective study of their value and current recommendations are based mainly upon empirical observation. Further research is needed to expand our knowledge and to increase the interest of health professionals.

1 Hunt A. *The elderly at home. A study of people aged sixty five and over living in the community in England in 1976.* London: OPCS, HMSO, 1978.
2 Moy A. *Aids assessment programme. Assessment of adult cutlery.* London: Department of Health and Social Security, 1985.
3 Wainwright H. Feeding problems in elderly disabled patients. *Nursing Times* 1978;**74**:542–3.
4 Mackenzie L, Aitken CA. Help in the home. Needs of disabled people. *British Journal of Occupational Therapy* 1982;**45**:293–4.
5 Smith ME, Walton MS, Garraway WM. Use of aids and adaptations in a study of stroke rehabilitation. *Health Bull (Edinb)* 1981;**39**:97–106.
6 Saunders J. The consumers' viewpoint. 1. Rheumatoid arthritis. *British Journal of Occupational Therapy* 1981;**44**:352.

Appendix

Recommended reading for patients

Nichols P, Haworth R, Hopkins J. *Disabled: an illustrated manual of help and self-help.* Newton Abbot, Devon: David and Charles, 1981.

Multiple Sclerosis Society. *Helpful hints around the home for the multiple sclerosis patient.* London: Multiple Sclerosis Society, 1980.

Arthritis and Rheumatism Council. *Your home and your rheumatism; aids and gadgets in the home.* London: Arthritis and Rheumatism Council, 1985.

Kitchen aids

M J CONNOLLY, A S WILSON

Disabilities that cause problems in performing simple domestic tasks can occur at any age but are most common in elderly people. Of those aged 70–74 living at home, 7% are unable to cook a meal; this figure rises to 27% for those aged 85 and over. The proportions unable to open screw top bottles in these age groups are 8% and 24% respectively.[1] Such difficulties may cause great distress, obliging disabled people to rely on others for help or even to relinquish their homes and enter residential care.

Providing aids may make the difference between maintenance or loss of independence. Gadgets, however, are not always appropriate, and basic guidelines for providing aids merit repetition: obtain assessment by an occupational therapist; provide aids only when other coping strategies fail; supply aids that are simple and look as normal and attractive as possible.

Some problems may be solved by giving simple advice: rather than trying to pour hot water from a pan let the water cool first and then empty it with a jug; push heavy pans along work surfaces rather than trying to carry them; cook vegetables in a chip basket placed in the pan—the basket may then be used to strain the vegetables when cooked. The provision of a wheeled trolley can facilitate the moving of food and utensils within the kitchen or from room to room.

Food stabilisers and bottle, jar, and can openers

Sterilisers and openers are often particularly valuable to patients with only one useful arm. Spiked boards (fig 1) stabilise bread, vegetables, or meat for cutting, but care is needed to choose one without dangerously sharp spikes. Of the many bottle top and jar lid removers marketed only those that fix to work surfaces or

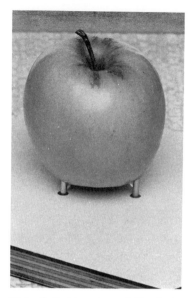

FIG 1—Spiked board to stabilise food for peeling or cutting

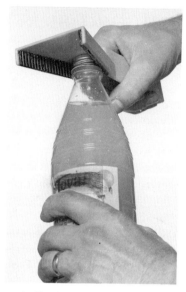

FIG 2—Bottle top remover

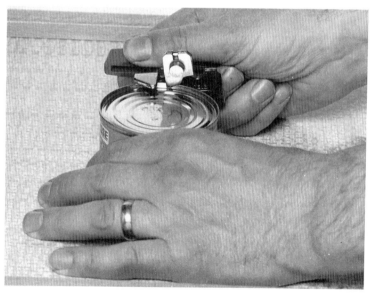

FIG 3—One handled tin opener

shelves are suitable for one handed people. Undoit and Skyline both need no adjustment, but while Undoit has a good serrated grip it is too small for large lids, whereas the larger, unserrated Skyline is too big for small lids. Both these devices need considerable pressure to wedge the jar or bottle into the "V".[2] Conventional wall mounted can openers need to be chosen carefully as some are difficult to operate if grip is weak whereas with others it is difficult to position the can in the mechanism.[2]

The aids and advice mentioned above may also apply when similar difficulties occur in patients with weakness, stiffness, pain, sensory loss, or tremor. In addition to wall mounted aids, however, a variety of hand held bottle, jar, and can openers are useful (figs 2–4). The Strongboy comprises a fulcrum and adjustable metal band that fits around the jar lid. Of all such devices it perhaps provides the greatest mechanical advantage and is suitable for those whose problem is weakness or pain, but adjustment of the band is difficult for those with tremor or lack of coordination.[2] The Twister (fig 5) is a conical rubber device needing no adjustment. It does, however, require heavy downward pressure and is therefore unsuitable if grip is poor. Patients whose main problem is lack of coordination find it the most helpful. In addition to wall mounted models, butterfly can openers with large knobs and handles are often suitable. Electrically operated openers can be helpful, though some are heavy.[2] Of the various jar stabilisers on the market, Spill Not is the simplest, needing no adjustment, but jars sometimes stick in its base.[3]

Knives

Knives, vegetable peelers, and other utensils with lightweight, large diameter handles are easier for those with poor grip. The Gustavasberg kitchen knives have large hand-saw handles, permitting a straight wrist (sawing motion) when cutting, with great mechanical advantage. Electric knives are heavy and often unsuitable.[3] The Ritter and PPL vegetable peelers have wide grip handles,[2] but an alternative for these (and indeed all knives and similar utensils) is to attach foam rubber plastazoate handles to conventional devices. Many patients with weak or painful hands have difficulty opening scissors, a problem overcome by selecting spring operated models.[3]

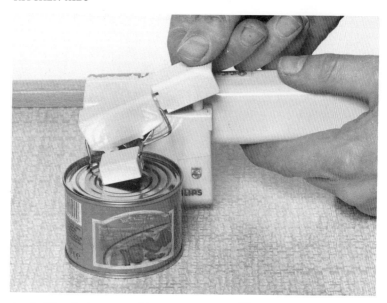

FIG 4—Electric tin opener with magnet to remove lid

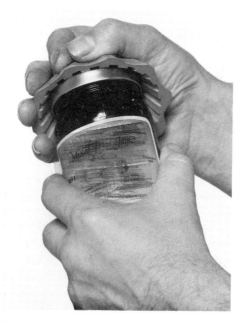

FIG 5—Twister

Food processors

Food processors and mixers are a great boon to many disabled people. When choosing from conventional models prime considerations are simplicity, weight, and ease of assembly and operation of the on–off switch.[4] They are, however, expensive, and the simple measure of spinning a normal hand whisk between the palms is often effective. Hand whisks with a spring action, using up down motion (spring whips) are valuable if shoulder movement is limited.[5]

Miscellaneous

Handiplugs (fig 6) ease difficulties inserting and removing electric plugs, and attachments to taps and cooker knobs make them easier to turn. Teapot tippers and kettle tippers (fig 7) obviate the need to lift heavy containers full of hot fluids, though kettle tippers should be (but are not) taller than the teapot tippers to facilitate teapot filling. Cup sized electric elements (originally designed for the use of travellers) may be more acceptable. A useful tip for those with poor reach or difficulty in bending is to use wax tapers instead of matches to light gas ovens or grills. Eye level grills, though easier to see, may be dangerous for disabled people to reach up to. Perching stools enable the user to sit at standing height for long periods without risk of toppling backwards. Microwave cookers may allow disabled people to prepare their own meals more easily (they can often be positioned more accessibly than conventional ovens and rings and they reduce cooking time) or allow them to reheat meals prepared by others. For those with visual impairment large bright utensils may be valuable, and alarms that bleep when a cup or pan is filled to preset levels might be considered.

Cognitive impairment poses specially difficult problems in preparing food. When moderate or severe it is not amenable to modification by aids, but when mild colour coded knobs may help safe use of a cooker as may timers with alarms. The simple provision of a whistle may prevent kettles burning dry. The increasing provision of the frozen meals service, which in many areas is replacing daily hot meal deliveries, may cause problems in heating the meal for moderately demented people. Microwaves are not usually appropriate here and may cause more trouble than benefit as confused elderly people may try to cook eggs or foil wrapped meals in them.

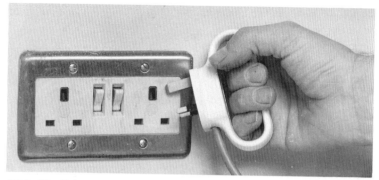

FIG 6—Handiplug

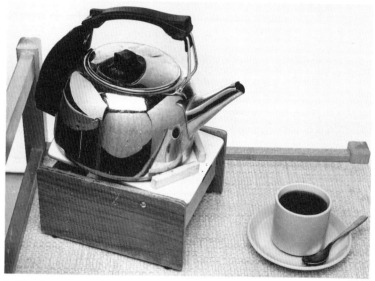

FIG 7—Kettle tipper for controlling pouring, useful for patients with tremor or poor grip

Conclusion

Detailed assessment and advice on availability and suitability of kitchen aids can be obtained from hospital or community based occupational therapists or from disabled living centres. Given the prevalence of disability in the kitchen in otherwise fit elderly people living at home it might be appropriate for kitchen assessments or predischarge home visits, common in geriatric units, to be extended to other specialties. Many problems that disabled people experience in the kitchen result from bad design. As so many people cannot open screw top jars or cans should we not be trying to design better food containers?

1 Hunt A. *The elderly at home. A study of people aged sixty five and over living in the community in England in 1976.* London: OPCS, HMSO 1978.
2 McIntosh R. *Aids assessment programme: food preparation aids for those with neurological conditions.* London: Department of Health and Social Security, 1983.
3 Bradshaw ESR. *Aids assessment programme. Food preparation aids for rheumatoid arthritis. 2A. Kitchen knives, scissors.* London: Department of Health and Social Security, 1985.
4 Bradshaw ESR. *Aids assessment programme. Food preparation aids for rheumatoid arthritis. 2B. Food choppers, graters, food processors.* London: Department of Health and Social Security, 1985.
5 Bradshaw ESR. *Aids assessment programme. Food preparation aids for rheumatoid arthritis. 2C. Whisks, hand held blenders, electric mixers.* London: Department of Health and Social Security, 1985.

Appendix

Recommended reading for patients

Nichols P, Haworth R, Hopkins J. *Disabled: an illustrated manual of help and self-help.* Newton Abbot, Devon: David and Charles, 1981.
Multiple Sclerosis Society. *Helpful hints around the home for the multiple sclerosis patient.* London: Multiple Sclerosis Society, 1980.
Arthritis and Rheumatism Council. *Your home and your rheumatism: aids and gadgets in the home.* London: Arthritis and Rheumatism Council, 1985.

Leisure and recreation

E WHITE

Many hobbies and pastimes may be enjoyed by disabled people, and being disabled should not mean being inactive or bored. Unfortunately, participating in a sport or pastime is often restricted as much by environmental barriers and unimaginative attitudes as by the disability itself.

Aids and appliances described in this and the previous series (such as splints and wheelchairs) may enable disabled people to take full advantage of the many leisure opportunities available. In addition to identifying what disabled people can and cannot do, it is most important to know what they find interesting and enjoyable. For many activities all that is needed is enthusiasm, for others it is usually a matter of finding alternative ways of doing something rather than designing new equipment. If a disabled person is unable to enjoy a particular leisure activity despite the provision of conventional aids, non-standard aids may be the answer. The Disabled Living Foundation may be able to help; often a solution to an individual problem has already been found. If a suitable aid is not available the Rehabilitation Engineering Movement Advisory Panel (a part of the Royal Association for Disability and Rehabilitation) has volunteer engineers and other staff who can design or adapt one off aids.

Access

A British Standards Institution code of practice covers requirements for access, and legislation now requires provision for needs of disabled people in public buildings and many new premises. Guides on access to various towns and areas are available from the Royal Association for Disability and Rehabilitation, which also produces the *Spectators' Access Guide for Disabled People.*

The National Trust's handbook indicates properties suitable for wheelchair users, and *The National Trust—Facilities for Disabled and Handicapped Visitors* gives further information. The English Heritage guide also lists properties with wheelchair access, and a separate guide gives more details, such as the number of steps.

The National Key Scheme provides access to special lavatories specifically for use by disabled people; there are many of these throughout the country, and a key and list are available from Royal Association for Disability and Rehabilitation or local social services departments.

Facilities for the disabled in public and historic buildings are slowly improving, but it is still wise to inquire in advance about provision for people with a specific disability.

Aids for leisure activities

Many games, such as chess, backgammon, and draughts, have been adapted for the blind, and the adapted versions are available from the Royal National Institute for the Blind. Playing cards for the visually impaired are also available. Card holders for those with difficulty holding the cards can be obtained, but a scrubbing brush will often serve as well (fig 1). Many games are available on microcomputer, and a joystick or other adapted control can enable disabled people to play individually or compete with others, including able bodied competitors.

Cinemas, theatres, and similar places can greatly help people with impaired hearing by installing induction loops as most hearing aids have a T setting.

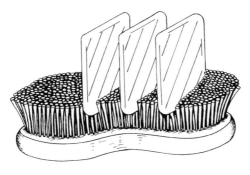

FIG 1—Scrubbing brush used to hold playing cards

Gardening

Gardening is one of the most popular recreational activities in Britain. It is important to consider the general design of the garden, such as the width of the beds, use of raised beds (fig 2), and layout of paths (fig 3). Many garden tools, though not sold specifically for disabled people, are designed to reduce physical effort—for example, by having longer handles to reduce bending. *Gardening*, a book in the series *Equipment for the Disabled*, has information on topics such as garden design, safety, and weeding; a range of tools is illustrated, and it also has a section on gardening for those with visual impairment. The Royal National Institute for the Blind produces a booklet (also in braille and on audiotape) *Gardening without Sight*, and the Society for Horticultural Therapy offers advice and help both to individual disabled gardeners and to professionals concerned with horticulture as a therapeutic activity.

Sport

The potential of disabled sportsmen and women was well demonstrated in the para-Olympics at Seoul; many sports may be adapted to take account of a disability—such as wheelchair basketball—and sport can offer an individual challenge no matter what the degree of disability. The British Sports Association for the Disabled promotes sport among disabled people and strives to improve facilities. Many bodies representing individual sports or disabilities can also help.

Angling is said to be the most popular participating sport in this country, and the Handicapped Piscatorial Association offers an advice service on all aspects of the sport and provides information on aids and equipment for the disabled. It also has a specially designed boat (Wheelyboat (fig 4)) which allows easy access for disabled people, including those in wheelchairs, and these are available at various locations throughout Great Britain.

Children's toys and play

Play is a vital part of a child's development, through which physical and social skills are learnt and practised. In general, standard toys should be provided for disabled children, together with the range of household items most children adopt for their

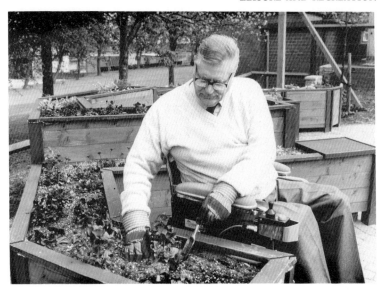

FIG 2—Raised flower beds. (Reproduced courtesy of William Merritt Disabled Living Centre, Leeds)

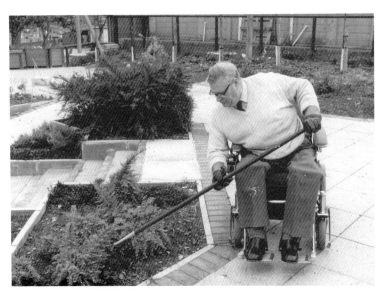

FIG 3—Garden designed for the disabled. (Reproduced courtesy of William Merritt Disabled Living Centre, Leeds)

63

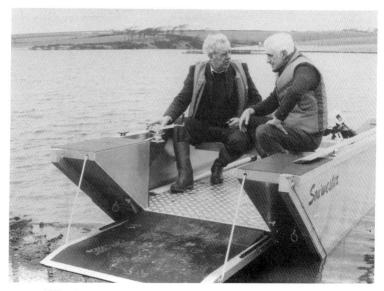

FIG 4—"Wheelyboat." (Reproduced courtesy of Handicapped Piscatorial Association)

play. Help and advice may be needed from the physiotherapist about posture and balance. Special chairs can be used to help support the child; these usually have an attached table at which the child can play. Many towns now have toy libraries, where a range of well tested toys may be borrowed. Play Matters (the National Toy Libraries Association) gives details of local libraries and also publishes *What Toy*.

Holidays

Many tour operators now offer facilities for disabled people in their standard packages. It is important to check early that they can accommodate people with specific disabilities. *Holidays for the Physically Handicapped*, published annually by the Royal Association for Disability and Rehabilitation, contains much detailed information on suitable accommodation. Other bodies, such as the Automobile Association, also produce helpful guides. Many activity holidays are available at special centres (for example, the Queen Elizabeth II Silver Jubilee Activities Centre, Hampshire), which offer residential activity courses for people who are mentally or physically disabled. Organisations that cater for people with specific disabilities run holidays themselves or can offer advice. Local social services departments may offer financial help with holidays for registered disabled people, but the amount varies greatly among districts. In the case of severely handicapped children aged under 16 and living at home the family fund, a government financed fund administered by the Joseph Rowntree Memorial Trust, may be able to provide financial help.

Obtaining help

A wealth of information and help is available. Most hobbies, sports, and pastimes have national representative bodies which provide information for disabled enthusiasts. There are also organisations specifically for physically and mentally disadvantaged people, many of which are listed in the *Directory for Disabled People*, which also includes self help groups. The Disabled Living Foundation has information notes on leisure activities and sports and physical recreation (information list numbers 6 and 6a) with addresses of helpful organisations. Disabled living centres can also offer specialist advice, and libraries and sports centres can help with information about local clubs. Information is also available from Disablement Information and Advice Lines, an independent advice service run by people with direct personal experience of disability.

Appendix

Further reading

British Standards Institute. *Access for the disabled in buildings.* BSI, 1979. (BS 5810.)

Cochrane GM, Wilshere ER, eds. *Gardening.* Oxford: Oxfordshire Health Authority, 1987. Available from Mary Marlborough Lodge, Nuffield Orthopaedic Centre, Oxford OX3 7ZD.

Corrado OJ. Hearing aids. In: Mulley G, ed. *Everyday aids and appliances.* London: British Medical Journal, 1989:1–8.

Darnborough A, Kinrade D. *Directory for disabled people: a handbook of information and opportunities for disabled and handicapped people.* 5th ed. Cambridge: Woodhead-Faulkner, 1989. Available in most main libraries for reference.

Chamberlain MA. Disabled living centres. In: Mulley G, ed. *Everyday aids and appliances.* London: British Medical Journal, 1989:96–101.

Jay P. *Coping with disability*. London: Disabled Living Foundation, 1984.
Thomson N, ed. *Sports and recreation provision for disabled people*. London: Disabled Living Foundation, 1984.

Addresses

British Sports Association for the Disabled, 34 Osnaburgh Street, London NW1 3ND (071 383 7277).

Disabled Living Foundation, 380–384 Harrow Road, London W9 2HU (071 289 6111). The Disabled Living Foundation will provide the address of your local Disabled Living Centre, which provides helpful advice on equipment for disability.

Disablement Information and Advice Lines (DIAL) UK, DIAL House, 117 High Street, Clay Cross, Derbyshire S45 9D2 (local addresses supplied).

English Heritage, Fortress House, 23 Savile Row, London W1Y 1AB.

Handicapped Piscatorial Association, 29 Ironlatch Avenue, St Leonards on Sea, East Sussex TN38 9JE (0424 427931).

Joseph Rowntree Memorial Trust, PO Box 50, York YO1 1UY.

National Trust, 36 Queen Anne's Gate, London SW1H 9AS.

Play Matters (the National Toy Libraries Association), 68 Churchway, London NW1 1CT (071 387 9592).

Queen Elizabeth II Silver Jubilee Activities Centre, Upper Hamble Country Park, Pylands Lane, Burlesden, Hampshire.

Rehabilitation Engineering Movement Advisory Panels (REMAP) and Royal Association for Disability and Rehabilitation (RADAR), 25 Mortimer Street, London W1N 8AB (071 637 5400).

Royal National Institute for the Blind (RNIB), 224 Great Portland Street, London W1N 6AA (071 388 1266).

Society for Horticultural Therapy, Goulds Ground, Vallis Way, Frome, Somerset BA11 3DW (0373 64782).

Appliances

Breast prostheses

JACQUELINE LEE

Every year 25 000 women in the United Kingdom are diagnosed as having breast cancer and for many the primary treatment will be surgery. It is important, therefore, that women are aware that after complete or even partial loss of a breast their natural shape can be restored by an artificial breast form known as a breast prosthesis. Women used to put a bag of birdseed or lentils inside their brassières (fig 1). Nowadays most breast prostheses are made of silicone, tinted to an appropriate shade and placed into preshaped bags of polyurethane, then placed into moulds and "baked" to gel the silicone to a consistency similar to normal breast tissue.

Types of prostheses

Many different brands are available and almost all can be obtained free of charge if the operation was performed under the NHS. If the operation was performed privately the prosthesis must be purchased (a list of stockists can be obtained from the Breast Care and Mastectomy Association). The cost of prostheses can vary between £70 and £170. Certain insurance schemes make an allowance towards this cost, so inquiries should be made. Most manufacturers carry four or five different shapes and up to 40 different sizes throughout their ranges. Because almost all are available free under the NHS, in theory every patient should be provided with a suitable prosthesis. The appliance officer in the hospital will be happy to give helpful advice about breast prostheses to patients as well as to health professionals.

Immediately after the operation a lightweight pad filled with fibre or foam and covered with cotton can be placed inside the bra. This can also be worn subsequently with nightwear. Later a permanent silicone prosthesis is provided (fig 2).

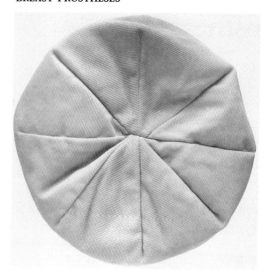

FIG 1—Early prosthesis: a bag of birdseed

For women who have had a partial mastectomy there are partial prostheses: soft, thin silicone shells that can restore the natural contour of the breast. When a lumpectomy has been performed a silicone wedge can be worn to good effect. These too are available in different sizes and free of charge under the NHS.

Several types of prostheses are available for use after simple mastectomy. Round prostheses (fig 3) are available in many sizes and are supplied with washable cotton covers. Women who have undergone more extensive surgery may use a heart shaped model (fig 4) or forms that taper gently to a round edge (fig 5). The shape and comfort of the woman are paramount in choosing the right prosthesis.

Silicone breast prostheses feel life-like and are long lasting. The polyurethane outer skin is completely impermeable: the patient can therefore swim in chlorinated water or the sea. Special swimwear and bras are available for women who have had breast surgery. These have retaining pockets to hold the prosthesis firmly in place while allowing a full range of movement. It is not always necessary to buy special bras, but choosing the correct size is important—many women tend to wear bras that are too small.

For educational purposes, training prostheses are available in a variety of models. They range from the type that contains multiple lumps to simulate fibrocystic conditions to one that contains enlarged ancillary nodes.

70

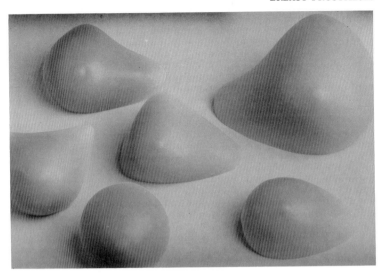

FIG 2—Variety of silicone prostheses. (Reproduced courtesy of Amoena (UK) Ltd)

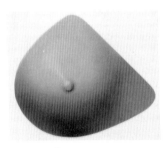

FIG 3—Breast form with nipple. (Reproduced courtesy of Anita Advisory Service)

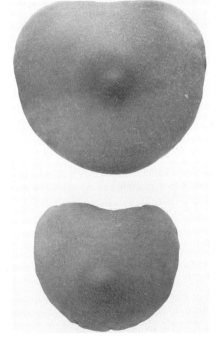

FIG 4—Heart shaped models (with washable cover). (Reproduced courtesy of Spenco Medical (UK) Ltd)

71

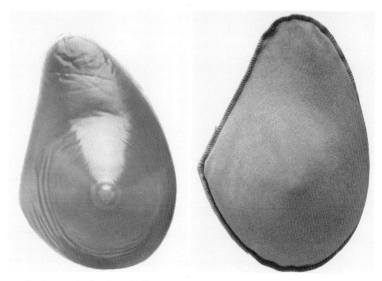

FIG 5—Anatomically shaped silicone breast form without and with cover. (Reproduced courtesy of Spencer of Banbury Ltd)

Fitting and provision

The fitting of the permanent prosthesis should ideally take place about six to eight weeks after the operation if the scar has healed well, or a little longer if radiotherapy is given. Most prostheses are guaranteed for between one and three years. A replacement prosthesis can be provided if the original one is damaged or if the size of the other breast has changed. A woman needing a new prosthesis who no longer attends a hospital for check ups or has moved to a new area will be referred by her general practitioner to a consultant surgeon, who will write a prescription, preferably worded "prosthesis to suit." She may then choose a suitable prosthesis from a range that should be available to view and try on either at the hospital or at an NHS approved stockist. The prosthesis will be fitted by either a breast nurse specialist, the hospital's appliance officer, or a fitter from a manufacturer.

A good fitter will give all the assistance he or she can, neither rushing nor pushing a person into making an incorrect choice. The psychological problems generated by a badly fitting or wrongly shaped prosthesis can be extremely damaging. Every day the woman is troubled by the discomfort and insecurity that the wrong prosthesis can cause: she never gets a chance to forget. She may take to wearing baggy clothes that are unflattering to her or make excuses to avoid social occasions. The wrong prosthesis is of no benefit in helping a woman get back to normal after breast surgery. Even obtaining the correct one can be a traumatic experience, so that some women opt to buy a prosthesis privately although they are fully entitled to receive one, free of charge, under the NHS.

Shortcomings in the provision of breast prostheses

The Breast Care and Mastectomy Association, reviewing 18 918 contacts in 1988, found that satisfaction with the fitting and provision of breast prostheses by the NHS orthotics service was low. There were six main complaints: no choice—patients were shown only one or two prostheses; not enough time taken during the fitting procedure; poor premises, no privacy, no mirror available (this caused great distress); delayed provision, some women having to wait up to six weeks after fitting for the prosthesis; being fitted by a man, although most male fitters themselves believe that fitting breast prostheses should be an exclusively female role; and the attitude of the fitter—nearly 70% of women thought that this was the most important consideration. When patients were asked which factor was the most important to them—choice, speed of provision, fitting location, or fitter—61% gave the attitude of the fitter as their top priority (M Baum and G Simpson, unpublished data).

Considerable publicity is rightly given to screening for breast cancer. It is regrettable that rather less thought and consideration is sometimes applied to the fitting and provision of breast prostheses.

Appendix

Useful addresses

Breastcare and Mastectomy Association, 26a Harrison Street, London WC1 8JG (071 837 0908); and 9 Castle Terrace, Edinburgh EH1 2DP (031 228 6715). A source of advice and information for any woman who has had breast surgery. Free leaflets available.

British Association of Cancer United Patients and their families and friends (BACUP), 121–123 Charterhouse Street, London EC1M 6AA (071 608 1661). Cancer information service. Booklets and leaflets on the practical and emotional aspects of coping with cancer.

Cancerlink, 17 Britannia Street, London WC1X 9JN (071 833 2451). Provides information on all aspects of cancer for people with cancer, their families and friends, and health professionals working with them.

Health Education Company, 12 Liverpool Terrace, Worthing, West Sussex BN11 1TA (0903 213694). Provides training prostheses for educational purposes.

Contact lenses

C STEVEN BAILEY, ROGER J BUCKLEY

Although public awareness of contact lenses seems to be increasing, the number of people wearing them remains uncertain. A population survey in 1988 indicated that about 4% of the population of the United Kingdom aged between 16 and 60 were wearing lenses regularly—that is, about 2·32 million people. Most wearers have lenses for cosmetic reasons; they are usually people with mild ametropia who prefer not to wear spectacles.

A smaller number of people are unable to attain satisfactory vision with glasses and can see adequately only with the aid of contact lenses. This group tends to be managed from hospital contact lens units and includes people with the following conditions.

- *Severe ametropia*—In very long or short sighted people spectacles are mechanically and optically unacceptable
- *Severe anisometropia*—Patients would experience intolerable aniseikonia with glasses. This group includes patients with unilateral aphakia
- *Severe regular astigmatism*—Patients experience disorientation and visual distortion with spectacles. The group includes patients with residual postoperative astigmatism, such as may occur after corneal transplantation
- *Irregular astigmatism*—In patients with this condition chaotic unevenness of the anterior corneal surface causes distortion of the ocular image. A rigid contact lens presents a smooth spherical anterior surface and the irregularity of the corneal surface behind the lens is filled in with tears. The lens may also mechanically flatten a thinned and distorted cornea. Patients with corneal ectasias, such as keratoconus, and corneal scarring fall into this category, as do some who have had corneal transplantation.

In addition, some people wear coloured lenses to disguise damaged and unsightly eyes. Corneoscleral, hard corneal, and soft lenses can have a hand painted pattern laminated into their substance. Soft lenses can also be made with a printed coloured pattern or with a homogeneous tint; both tend to sacrifice realism for economy. All such lenses may be powered for vision if required. Finally, therapeutic lenses may be needed to protect a diseased ocular surface.

Types of contact lenses

Scleral lenses

Contact lenses were first clinically described by Fick in 1888[1] and Muller in 1889.[2] These early corneoscleral shells and lenses were blown in glass: a central lens vaulted the cornea and the peripheral skirt was supported by the sclera. The modern equivalents of these "scleral" or "haptic" lenses were made possible by the discovery of Perspex in 1934. Even though tear exchange behind such lenses can be facilitated by fenestrations, channels, or slots (fig 1), considerable hypoxic and metabolic stresses are placed on the cornea, which usually result in changes such as peripheral vascularisation and endothelial cell abnormality in the long term. Sclerlal lenses are nevertheless invaluable for managing extreme degrees of ametropia and astigmatism that cannot be corrected with corneal lenses. Their large size makes for easy handling, which can benefit people with poor dexterity. Furthermore, recent experiments in their manufacture with modern gas permeable materials promises a much wider application in the future. Because of the special skills needed to make scleral lenses, the time involved, and the consequent high cost, they are rarely fitted except in a few hospital contact lens units.

Perspex hard lenses

The lenses commonly in use today are described as hard corneal (hard, rigid) or soft (fig 2). The first hard lens was introduced in 1947 and was later developed into corneal microlenses of up to 9.5 mm in diameter. This type of lens was made from perspex and continues to be used today in various modified forms. Perspex has a negligible maximum water content of 0.2% to 0.4% and is virtually impermeable to oxygen. Gas exchange with the corneal

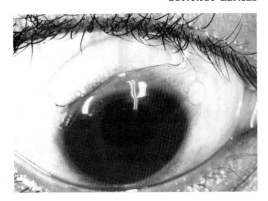

FIG 1—Scleral lens with fenestration at top to aid tear flow under lens

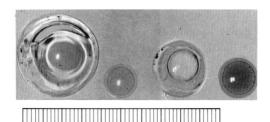

FIG 2—Types of contact lenses. *From left to right*: scleral, Perspex (rigid), hydrogel (soft), and gas permeable rigid lenses

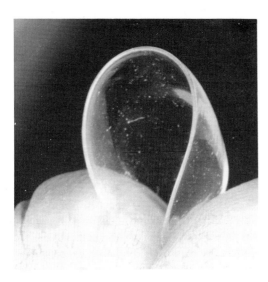

FIG 3—Hydrogel lens flexed between finger and thumb

epithelium is therefore dependent on tears flowing behind the lens. To ensure that the central corneal surface is adequately supplied with oxygen the lens must be made quite small. Its posterior surface is formed into a curve, which allows good movement on the cornea and encourages tear exchange.

Soft lenses

Because Perspex lenses can be difficult to fit and may not be well tolerated the introduction of the hydrogel soft lens in the late 1960s represented an important advance (fig 3). The first lenses were made from polyhydroxyethylmethacrylate, although their modern descendants are cross linked with other compounds to improve their physical properties. The water content of soft lenses varies from 35% to 80%. Soft lenses are cheaper to produce and are much easier to fit than Perspex or gas permeable hard ones; they are comfortable from the start, and, because the user does not need to build up tolerance to them, they can be useful for occasional wear. On the debit side they are costly: they tend to be expensive to buy, and they usually require more money to be spent on solutions to care for them than do other lenses. They are far less durable than rigid lenses and require much more frequent replacement. A good life for a soft lens disinfected by chemical means might be 12 to 18 months. Lenses that are disinfected by heat may last as little as six months.

Unlike a rigid lens, which can nullify some degree of corneal astigmatism by presenting a spherical surface to the atmosphere, a soft lens wraps on to the cornea and conforms to its curvature. Ordinary soft lenses are therefore unable to correct more than a slight corneal astigmatism. Soft lenses with a toric anterior surface can be fitted to people with astigmatism (fig 4) but they are expensive and may not always provide stable vision because of their tendency to rotate on the eye. To stabilise them they may have to be ballasted, and this can produce a thick inferior edge. The lower part of the cornea can then become starved of oxygen with consequent vascularisation. Very thick lenses, which do not follow fine irregularities of the corneal surface well, can be used to correct the irregular astigmatism of keratoconus and scarring, but they induce substantial metabolic stresses and consequently enhance the hazards of long term wear.

Because they are permeable to oxygen, soft lenses can be made much larger than rigid Perspex ones: typically 12·5 mm or more in

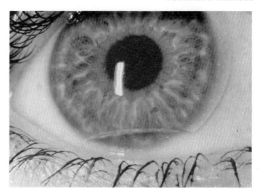

FIG 4—Toric hydrogel lens on eye, truncated at inferior edge to prevent excessive rotation

diameter. A large lens gives better vision than a small one as it centres well and can have a large optical zone. The larger lens is also more comfortable because it is less mobile and its edges are behind the lid margins and so do not impact on them during blinking. Unfortunately, the long circumference tends to irritate the tarsal conjunctiva and the high surface area maximises the deposition of potentially antigenic substances.

Gas permeable lenses

The problems of correcting astigmatism with soft lenses led manufacturers to seek other gas permeable materials that would combine the advantages of both Perspex and polyhydroxyethyl-methacrylate; both the mechanical rigidity of the hard lens and the gas permeability of the soft one were important. The first hard gas permeable material used was cellulose acetate butyrate in 1937. Unfortunately, the optical quality was poor and the material fell into disuse until the 1970s, when incentive and improved manufacturing techniques produced a renewed surge of interest. Cellulose acetate butyrate has a maximum water content of only 2·2%, and, like other hard gas permeable materials, it therefore depends on its chemical structure to pass oxygen across its molecular lattice-work. More modern materials, which incorporate substances such as silicone and fluorine into their structure, now easily outperform soft lenses in their ability to transmit oxygen. Gas permeable devices (fig 5) are therefore less liable to induce metabolic stresses than are hydrogels.

As the surface area is smaller than for a soft lens and the tendency of most hard gas permeable materials to attract deposits

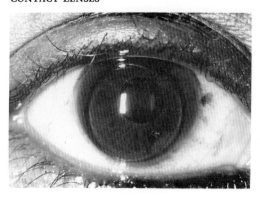

FIG 5—Rigid gas permeable lens on eye. Lens is engraved R to help wearer distinguish it from left one

is less than that of hydrogels the risk of deposit related problems is reduced. Because the material is gas permeable a larger lens can be tolerated than would be the case if the lens were made of Perspex. The movement of the lens and its impact velocity on the lid edge is therefore less than for a small hard lens, making the gas permeable lens more comfortable.

Although they are not as rigid as Perspex lenses, hard gas permeable lenses are sufficiently inflexible to correct similar degrees of corneal astigmatism. These modern lenses still require expensive solutions to maintain them but cost less to maintain than soft lenses. Gas permeable lenses are more easily damaged than Perspex ones, but they can still give up to two years of service before microscopic structural changes occur because of mechanical and chemical degradation.

In a comparison of instantaneous comfort the soft lens wins and may be tolerated for a full day's wear from the start. In contrast, to reach a continuous wear time of 10 hours with a Perspex lens may take several weeks of gradually increasing the number of hours during which the lens is worn each day. With a highly gas permeable lens the same wear time can often be achieved in five days.

Another lens material, which lies between the hard and soft groups, is silicone rubber. This has a high gas permeability, and its optical properties are excellent. Being soft yet containing no water, it may be suitable for fitting to tear deficient eyes. Its surface is hydrophobic, however, and the lenses have a tendency to collect deposits badly despite attempts to reduce this by surface coating; this has limited their use to special applications in hospital contact lens units.

Care of contact lenses

Lenses worn only during waking hours are cleaned and disinfected after removal every day. The cleaning process removes the environment derived and tear related deposits and breaks down the microbial biofilm, which collect during wear. Both surfaces are treated with a special fluid, which is usually specific to each type of lens material (fig 6). The cleaning solution should then be rinsed off before the lenses are soaked overnight in fresh disinfecting solution. This is because the cleaning solution can reduce the effectiveness of the disinfectant. The lenses may be rinsed again before being reinserted. Users of rigid lenses may prefer to apply a viscous cushioning solution (known as a wetting solution) to their lenses immediately before placing them on their eyes. Only sterile isotonic saline sold in pressurised canisters must be used to rinse soft lenses. (Sterile isotonic saline is also available in unit dose sachets, but these are less convenient and economical.)

It is probably expedient to rinse cleaning fluid off rigid lenses with rising main tap water (depending on its quality) as they will subsequently be placed in a disinfecting solution, but plain tap water must not be applied to the lenses after they have been disinfected. If tap water is used between the cleaning and disinfecting processes it may be wise to rinse this off with a brief

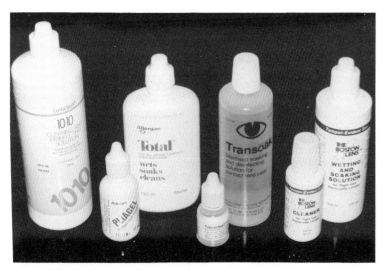

FIG 6—Selection of contact lens care solutions

application of sterile saline or freshly boiled and cooled tap water. Soft lenses may be disinfected by heat, which saves on solutions but shortens the life of the lens and tends to make protein deposits more difficult to remove.

Among the alternative cold chemical solutions 3% hydrogen peroxide is probably the most effective. Contrary to some manufacturers' current recommendations, however, it is still necessary to clean the lenses before disinfection. Also, although a 10 minute disinfection cycle may be specified in the instructions, a soaking time of at least two hours is now known to be necessary to eliminate acanthamoeba trophozoites and cysts (RE Silvary *et al*, Contact Lens Association of Ophthalmologists and International Society of Refractive Keratoplasty annual meeting, New Orleans, 1989) and overnight soaking is recommended. Only hydrogen peroxide solutions that are specifically formulated for contact lenses must be used, and solutions must be neutralised with the additional unit dose unpreserved solutions provided before the lenses are reworn. The system that uses a platinum disc to catalyse the degradation of the peroxide during the disinfection process cannot be recommended because it has inadequate antiacanthamoebal activity.

Almost all soft lens wearers, and some wearers of gas permeable lenses, will need to treat their lenses with proteolytic enzymes every few weeks. Protein removal is carried out as an extra stage after cleaning the lenses and before disinfecting them. The enzyme tablets are dissolved in sterile isotonic saline, and the lenses are soaked for a period which varies according to the type of lens and the particular enzymatic product. It is best to clean and rinse the lenses again afterwards, before disinfecting them, as the enzymes may only loosen the deposits and a mechanical action is desirable to complete their removal.

Every lens case must be cleaned weekly with hot water and a small brush, such as a toothbrush intended for children. Soap and detergents should not be used. After rinsing with rising main tap water the case should be shaken to remove surplus water, its outside blotted with a tissue, and then left to air dry before its next use. Cases should be discarded and replaced as soon as they have become discoloured or deposited, or whenever the lenses are renewed. Because of the nature and sources of contact lens related keratitis, ornate and expensive permanent lens cases should not be used unless they have a replaceable inner component. No regimen for the extended wear (see glossary) of lenses can yet be said to be satisfactory.

Risks of lenses

Contact lenses are foreign bodies on the eye and may induce changes that can be sight threatening. Many studies have examined the complications associated with specific lens types and some have compared the risks of wearing different sorts of lenses. Few attempts have been made to determine the size of the problem of contact lens associated eye disease in a community, however, although a long term prospective study of people presenting with complications of cosmetic lenses is currently under way at Moorfields Eye Hospital.

Daily wear rigid lenses have been found to be the safest type and extended wear soft ones the most dangerous.[3-6] Schein et al showed that people who wear extended wear soft lenses day and night have as much as a 15 times higher risk of suppurative keratitis than do people who wear daily wear soft lenses only during the waking hours.[4] Furthermore, they also found that for users of extended wear lenses the risk of suppuration was incrementally related to the number of nights over which the lenses were worn. This indicates that the predisposing factors to suppuration are cumulative. If physiological stress is implicated it would seem that the eye is being progressively compromised without the opportunity for recovery. Extended wear of soft lenses seems to carry a 21 times greater risk of microbial keratitis compared with the daily wear of gas permeable rigid lenses.[7]

Although the exact amount of oxygen that the cornea requires to prevent measurable changes in its characteristics[8] (the critical oxygen requirement) is still debated,[9] clearly no hydrogel lens can meet these metabolic needs. Though some gas permeable materials show greater promise in this respect, the extended wear of contact lenses is presently dangerous, and its practice for cosmetic use cannot be condoned.

Perhaps we shall one day have sufficient understanding of the adverse mechanisms, and the technology appropriate for overcoming them, for the risks of extended wear to be reduced to those of daily wear. Until then overnight wear of soft lenses can be justified only in three instances. The first is for people who have a medical need for contact lenses but are unable to handle them. These include infants and some elderly people with aphakia and people with some specific disabilities. The second is for people who require therapeutic lenses for corneal disorders; but the danger of supplementing their disorder with an even more devastating one must be carefully considered. The third is for people living in hostile environments where it is deemed that removing the lenses for cleaning and disinfection is likely to be more hazardous than leaving them in place. Such people will usually need to wear their lenses for only a few nights before returning to daily wear. Only the last group is likely to present to high street optometric practices; the others should always be treated in hospital. All other patients should wear lenses only during waking hours.

Disposable soft contact lenses have recently been introduced. They are priced to be competitive for extended wear for periods of one to two weeks. Although they are claimed to promote eye health by eliminating the complications associated with lens deposition and reactions to lens care solutions, they are unlikely to be superior to reusable lenses in any other respect.[10] Alarming numbers of cases of suppurative keratitis are now being reported in association with disposable lenses, and practitioners should be aware that their use cannot be assumed to be beneficial until the results of proper epidemiological studies are available.

Overall, those who wish to wear their lenses for many hours on most days of the week should be fitted in a gas permeable rigid material, if possible. Daily wear soft lenses should be reserved for people who have only an occasional need for their lenses, who prove to be intolerant of rigid ones, or who have needs which cannot be met by rigid lenses.

Successful contact lens wear requires scrupulous attention to detail. The users must understand that it is vital that they conform to the recommended maintenance and wear regimens for the types of lens that they have. Complications are common, but it is unusual for serious disease to arise when lenses are used responsibly.

Most complications of contact lenses are self limiting if the lens is removed at the first hint of trouble. All wearers must be counselled to remove their lenses immediately and seek professional advice if they experience ocular pain, red eye, or visual loss. Topical drug treatment must not be instituted without removal of the lens, and topical steroids should be used only in specialist centres.

Contact lens practitioners should routinely give thorough instructions to patients on the proper handling and care of their lenses and should back this advice up with a written information. Routine progress checks are important to detect the more covert problems at an early stage. Twice yearly examinations are recommended for full time wearers of soft lenses and annual examinations for those with rigid lenses.

1 Fick AE. A contact lens. May C, transl. *Archives of Ophthalmology New York* 1988;**17**:215–6. (Eine Contactbrille. *Arch Augenheilkd* 1888;**18**:279.)
2 Pearson RM, Effron N. Hundredth anniversary of August Muller's inaugural dissertation on contact lenses. *Surv Ophthalmol* 1989;**34**:133–41.
3 Franks WA, Adams GGW, Dart JKG, Minassian D. Relative risks for different types of contact lenses. *BMJ* 1988;**297**:524–5.
4 Schein OD, Glynn RJ, Poggio EC, Seddon JM, Kenyon KR. The relative risk of ulcerative keratitis among users of daily wear and extended wear soft contact lenses. *N Engl J Med* 1989;**321**:773–8.
5 Poggio EC, Glynn RJ, Schein OD, Seddon JM, *et al.* The incidence of ulcerative keratitis among users of daily wear and extended wear soft contact lenses. *N Engl J Med* 1989;**321**:779–83.
6 Stapleton F, Dart JKG, Minassian D. The relative risks of different contact lenses. *Invest Ophthalmol Vis Sci* 1989;**30** (Suppl):166.
7 Stapleton F. *British Contact Lens Association continuing program of education—extended wear of contact lenses.* London:BCLA, 1990.
8 Efron N, Brennan NA. In search of the critical oxygen requirement of the cornea. *Contax* 1987 July:5.
9 Holden BA. Corneal requirements for extended wear: an update. *CLAO (New Orleans LA)* 1988;**14**:220.
10 Dart JKG. Disposable extended wear contact lenses. *Lancet* 1988;**i**:1437.

Glossary

Ametropia—A condition in which there is some error of refraction in consequence of which parallel rays, with the eyes' accommodation at rest, are not focused on the retina. May refer to myopia (short sight) or to hyperopia (long sight).

Anisometropia—A difference in the power of refraction of the two eyes.

Anisekonia—A relative difference in the size or shape of the images in the two eyes. Small differences can be tolerated by cerebral adaptation, but an image size difference of more than 10% will almost certainly result in double vision.

Aphakia—Absence of the crystalline lens, or a lens implant, after surgery for cataract. (If an implant lens is inserted the eye is said to be pseudophakic.)

Astigmatism—A condition of unequal curvatures along the different meridia at one or more of the refractive surfaces of the eye (here, that of the anterior cornea), in consequence of which the rays from a luminous point are not focused at a single point on the retina but are spread out as a line in one or another direction. Thus, if the person were viewing a cross the image of only one of the two arms could be focused on the retina at a time; the other would be focused in front or behind it, and would therefore appear blurred.

Regular astigmatism—The curvatures in each meridian are of different radii but follow the normal topography of the surface.

Irregular astigmatism—The radii of curvatures vary randomly because the surface is uneven.

Daily wear—The lenses are worn only during the waking hours and are removed before sleep.

Extended wear—The continuous wear of contact lenses throughout the waking and sleeping hours, without interruption.

Toric—Relating to, or having the curvature of, a torus (see below).

Torus—A geometrical figure formed by the revolution of a circle round the base of any of its arcs. The result is a smoothly contoured surface that has different radii of curvature in different meridia. In the case of a refractive surface such as the anterior surface of the cornea, the refractive power will be greatest for light incident perpendicular to the meridian of greatest curvature (smallest radius of curvature), and least for light falling perpendicular to the meridian of least curvature (largest radius of curvature).

Dentures

OLIVER J CORRADO

A quarter of all adults in Britain have no natural teeth. This proportion increases progressively with age to 65% of people aged 65–74 and 82% of those aged 75 and over.[1] Many people with partial or complete tooth loss can be helped by wearing dentures.

History

Fairly elaborate partial dentures were made by the Etruscans as early as 700 BC. Some were removable; others were fixed to neighbouring teeth. Subsequently, artificial teeth were made from ivory, wood, bone, silver, mother of pearl, enamelled copper, or porcelain. Even teeth from other humans have been used. Until the middle of the nineteenth century denture bases were generally made from gold or ivory, but these were superseded by vulcanite (rubber hardened with sulphur), which remained popular until the 1940s, when poly (methylmethacrylate) resin was used to construct teeth and bases. Some elderly people still possess vulcanite dentures—these can be recognised by their characteristic colours.

Classification of dentures

Dentures can be divided into two groups.[2] Complete dentures are designed to replace either the entire maxillary (upper) or mandibular (lower) dentitions. Most are made from acrylic resin but some incorporate metal palates (generally either cobalt-chromium alloy or stainless steel) when additional strength is required. Removable partial dentures are designed to replace missing teeth for partially edentulous patients and are made of acrylic resin or metal. Some are retained by physical forces such as adhesion and cohesion and by muscular control, but many incorporate mechani-

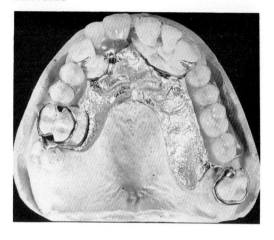

FIG 1—Partial denture incorporating metal (cobalt-chromium alloy) retainers. Denture is mounted on plaster model

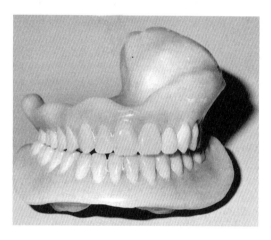

FIG 2—Complete dentures supplied for a patient after maxillary surgery. Upper denture includes obturator on left side

cal devices (retainers) for this purpose. These include clasps, studs, and more elaborate locking mechanisms (fig 1).

An overdenture (overlay denture) is a removable denture (partial or complete) that is fitted over retained, prepared roots or natural teeth. Partial dentures and overdentures can be used as an interim step before complete dentures are fitted, enabling patients to gradually adapt to denture wearing. Partial and complete dentures may have to be modified to include an obturator, which is an extension of the denture base designed to fill a congenital defect (for example, cleft palate) or one that has been acquired (for example, after operation) (fig 2). The obturator improves speech, masticatory function, and appearance.

The first set of complete dentures

Patients used to wait several months after tooth extraction before complete dentures were fitted. This allowed the tissues to heal and much of the alveolar bone to resorb. Nowadays most patients have complete dentures fitted at the same visit as their remaining natural teeth are extracted (immediate dentures). This method is advantageous because it maintains dental and facial appearances, reduces masticatory and speech disturbances, facilitates adaptation to dentures, and allows the appearance of the natural teeth to be copied. Patients have to be monitored closely after immediate dentures are fitted as modifications will often be required.

To make the dentures, impressions are taken, casts made, and the correct anatomical relation of the upper and lower jaws recorded and reproduced. Trial dentures are formed on the casts with the artificial teeth positioned in wax and these dentures are tried in the patient. Tooth selection is important: artificial teeth come in a variety of shades, shapes, and sizes, and their incisal edges and surfaces have varying degrees of smoothness and regularity. The shade should complement the skin or complexion, and the shape should be appropriate for the patient's sex, facial structure, personality, and body build. Most teeth are made of acrylic resin and are attached to the denture base by chemical union. Sometimes porcelain teeth attached to the base by pins are used: these are harder wearing, but may make more noise and chip more easily. Whichever material is used the arrangement should look natural: if too perfect, the teeth may appear artificial (fig 3). When the cosmetic appearance has been approved the trial dentures are processed in acrylic resin.

Patients with symptoms of recent onset who have an existing set of dentures that has given satisfactory service can have these copied; fairly minor changes in design can be made on the copies. This technique is particularly valuable for elderly patients, who might have great difficulty adapting to and controlling a totally new shape.

89

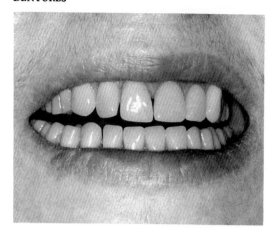

FIG 3—Variation in tooth alignment to create a more natural appearance in complete dentures

Information and follow up

Patients should be advised about oral hygiene and denture care at the time of fitting and also given written information about eating, cleaning, controlling, and possible problems.[3] Providing written information helps to prevent unnecessary difficulties. Recommendations regarding the review of patients fitted with dentures vary. Patients fitted with partial dentures and overdentures should be seen at intervals of about six months to monitor oral hygiene and to undertake regular maintenance of the remaining teeth and associated periodontal tissues. Immediate dentures often require early modification, and patients should be seen frequently over the first three months (for example, after 24 hours, one week, two weeks, one month, and three months) and annually thereafter. Patients with complete dentures should have a routine check every three to five years.

Patient satisfaction

The principal objectives in denture construction are that: facial appearance and shape should be restored and the artificial teeth should appear attractive and natural; the denture should be as well retained and as comfortable as the remaining oral structures allow; the denture should permit a satisfactory level of function; and the denture should not damage supporting tissues.

The patient's attitude greatly influences the success of dentures.[4]

Natural tooth loss may be associated with a mild grief reaction: this was found in half the wearers of complete dentures and more commonly in women than men.[4] Successful prosthetic treatment depends on good relationships between the patient, dental surgeon, and dental technician. With time 70% of patients accept complete dentures as part of themselves, and 75% feel awkward about being seen without them.[4] Many patients are quite satisfied with dentures that are judged by dental surgeons to be less than satisfactory. Equally, some patients have the greatest difficulty in accepting dentures that have been designed and constructed to the highest standards.

Denture problems

Systemic disease may predispose to denture problems. For example, diabetes is associated with an increased incidence of oral candidiasis. Xerostomia, which commonly occurs as a side effect of drug treatment, may make it more difficult to retain dentures and cause excessive mucosal irritation because of reduced salivary lubrication. Problems are more common with complete dentures. Sheppard *et al* found denture related oral lesions in almost half of patients.[5]

Pain is a common symptom in wearers of complete dentures and may be caused by small or large defects in denture design, problems in the denture bearing tissues, or as a consequence of systemic disease. Mandibular parafunction not infrequently contributes to the complaint. Patients should be encouraged to seek advice from their dental surgeon and must be discouraged from trying to treat themselves with "over the counter" products.

Loose dentures—Alveolar resorption occurs with time and causes dentures to lose their fit (fig 4). This happens much less commonly with the type of partial denture that is supported by the remaining natural teeth. The problem occurs most often in the lower edentulous jaw, which resorbs about four times faster than the upper. If the problem is related to the fitting surface of the denture the fit may be improved by relining or rebasing the denture. An immediate denture usually needs to be rebased in the first few months after the last teeth were extracted. As with the complaint of pain, the aetiology is diverse and correct treatment depends on an accurate diagnosis.

Denture stomatitis is an inflammatory condition affecting the oral mucosa covered by the denture. It occurs in up to 60% of denture wearers, is commoner in the upper jaw and in women, and is generally painless. The condition may be caused by infection (particularly candidiasis) or denture trauma and may be complicated by systemic problems. It is therefore important to establish the correct diagnosis so that appropriate treatment can be given. Where there is an infective component a fungicide is often unnecessary as the condition will often resolve when plaque on the denture surface is controlled with hypochlorite denture cleansing solution. Chemical irritation from mouthwashes, ointments, pastes, fixatives, and chemical constituents in the denture material may also cause stomatitis. Pain or discomfort is usually a component of stomatitis arising from these causes.

Angular stomatitis (cheilosis) is an erythematous condition of the angles of the mouth; it is usually bilateral (fig 5) and is often associated with an infective denture stomatitis. Creasing of the skin at the mouth angles, which is a contributory factor, may indicate poor lip support by the dentures, but this creasing may result from an age related loss of muscle tone.

Papillary hyperplasia—Irritation of the palatal mucosa by the denture may produce mucosal hyperplasia, which may be associated with denture stomatitis. Treatment should include denture hygiene and reducing denture trauma, sometimes by constructing a new denture with a smoother fitting surface. As for denture stomatitis, dentures should not be worn at night.

Denture trauma may produce bands of fibrous tissue, commonly in the labial sulci. This condition is often painful at first, and it may be associated with ulceration, but patients often put up with the discomfort and allow the trauma to produce the relatively painless hyperplasia. Poorly fitting dentures should be adjusted and occlusal abnormalities corrected. Excision of the tissue may be required, in which case the specimen should be sent to an oral pathologist for examination.

Excessive salivation and impaired speech—Excessive salivation may occur for a few days after a new denture has been fitted, but it will settle. Similarly, some difficulty with speech may be encountered until patients adapt to denture wearing; persisting speech disturbance needs to be investigated.

Chewing—The chewing efficiency of a wearer of complete dentures is about a fifth of that of people with natural dentition. Patients may encounter difficulty eating crisp foods such as apples,

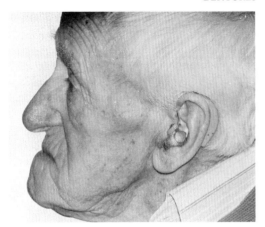

FIG 4—Altered facial appearance due to ill fitting complete dentures resulting in loss of facial height and protrusion of mandible

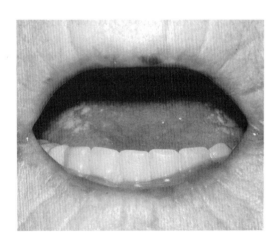

FIG 5—Angular stomatitis

and a third of wearers of complete dentures have to avoid certain foods. Patients with new dentures should be advised to cut food up into small pieces, to eat soft foods at first, and to distribute food equally on both sides of the mouth. As muscular control improves in the first few weeks, so does chewing efficiency.

Denture fixatives

Many denture wearers purchase fixatives to improve retention. Bates and Murphy found that a tenth of denture wearers had used these at some time.[6] Fixatives are available as powders, pastes, liquids, and adherent bandages[7]; common ingredients are karaya gum or tragacanth gum, which become gelatinous with water. Fixatives can help retain immediate or new dentures in the short term, help retain obturators, and aid denture retention when physiological factors are suboptimal—for example, when there is xerostomia.[7] Fixatives should not be used without professional advice because they may hide a problem that may lead to further resorption of the underlying bone.

Denture hygiene

Half of denture wearers clean their dentures inadequately (fig 6). Poor denture hygiene allows plaque to develop, leading to halitosis and predisposing to denture stomatitis. The problem is particularly important with partial dentures as plaque will lead to periodontal disease and dental caries. Dentures should be removed at night to let the oral tissues rest. Denture cleansers include alkaline hypochlorite solutions, alkaline peroxides available as soluble powders or tablets, acid solutions, antibacterial and enzymatic preparations, and pastes with varying abrasion. Hypochlorite solutions are highly effective at removing plaque and are probably the cleanser of choice,[2] but they may corrode metal.

Harrison has recommended the following cleaning procedure.[2] The denture should be brushed with a soft toothbrush and soap and water. This should be done over a full washbasin or bowl of water to reduce the chance of damage if the denture is dropped. Specially designed brushes are available which may be useful to those disabled or elderly people who have poor manual dexterity (figs 7 and 8). After rinsing the denture should be soaked in an alkaline hypochlorite solution overnight to reduce plaque; if the denture incorporates metal it should be immersed for no longer than 30 minutes in solution of the manufacturer's recommended dilution.

Denture identification

Identification marks allowing the wearer to be identified may be useful in coma, amnesia, major disasters, and for forensic purposes. Identification is also valuable in hospitals and other institutions if dentures are misplaced or lost temporarily. Ideally all

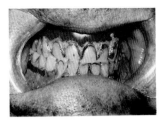

FIG 6—Extreme example of poor denture hygiene

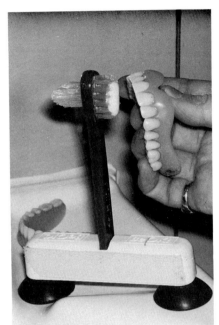

FIG 7—Suction denture brush

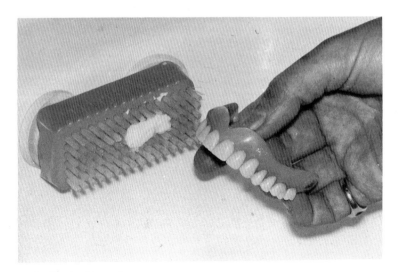

FIG 8—Brush with suction cups

95

dentures should be marked during construction, but in Britain this is done routinely only by the armed forces and by certain dental laboratories.

Identification marks (such as the patient's name) can be applied to the denture surface by hospital staff. The ideal marking system should be cheap, easy to perform, and durable and should not damage the denture. Identification marks can be written on the surface and then coated with a protective sealant. Marks made by spirit pens are not very durable. A commercial denture marking kit (see appendix) includes an abrasive pad to clean and roughen the surface of the denture, a marking pencil, and sealant; the marks remain legible for about six months.[2]

The loss of a set of dentures belonging to an elderly person is often a major problem. Advanced age and deteriorating health may make it impossible for the patient to learn to control new shapes. Providing replacement dentures is not a simple procedure. The message should be clear—prevention is better than cure.

I thank Professor RM Basker, professor of dental prosthetics and consultant in restorative dentistry, University of Leeds, for advice; Mr BR Nattress, lecturer in restorative dentistry, University of Leeds, for supplying figure 2; Miss Anna Paulin, senior occupational therapist, Leeds General Infirmary, for supplying figures 7 and 8; and the photographic departments of the Leeds General Infirmary and School of Dentistry.

1 Office of Population Censuses and Surveys. The 1983 update on adult dental health from OPCS. Br Dent J 1986;160:246–53.
2 Harrison A. Denture care. Nursing Times 1987;83:28–9.
3 Wendt DC. How to promote and maintain good oral health in spite of wearing dentures. J Prosthetic Dent 1985;53:805–7
4 Berg E, Ingebretsen R, Johnson TB. Some attitudes towards edentulousness, complete dentures and cooperation with the dentist. Acta Odontol Scand 1984;42:334–8
5 Sheppard IM, Schwartz LR, Sheppard SM. Oral status of edentulous and complete denture-wearing patients. J Am Dent Assoc 1971;83:614–20.
6 Bates JF, Murphy WM. A survey of an edentulous population. Br Dent J 1968;124:116–21.
7 Polyzois GL. An update on denture fixatives. Dental Update 1983;October: 579–83.

Appendix

Useful Information

Suction denture brushes and brushes with suction cups cost about £7.25 and £9.75 respectively (inclusive of VAT) and are available from the UK suppliers: AREMCO, Grove House, Lenham, Kent ME17 2PX (0622 858502).

Identure Marking Kits cost about £31.50 (including VAT). Information on local suppliers can be obtained from: Dental Products Group, 3M Health Care Ltd, 3M House, 1 Morley Street, Loughborough LE1 1EP (0509 611611).

Advice leaflets for denture wearers

Keep Smiling. Available from: The Product Manager, Household Toiletries Division, Reckitt and Colman, Reckitt's House, Stoneferry Road, Hull HU8 8BD (0482 26151).

Smile With Confidence. Available from: The Professional Relations Officer, Stafford-Miller House, The Common, Hatfield AL10 0NZ (0707 261151).

Further Reading

Basker RM, Davenport JC, Tomlin HR. *Prosthetic treatment of the edentulous patient*. London: Macmillan, 1983.

Woodforde J. *The strange story of false teeth*. London: Routledge and Kegan Paul, 1968.

Devlin H, Bedi R. Denture use and abuse. *Dental Update* 1988;March:78–80.

Abelson DC. Denture plaque and denture cleansers: review of the literature. *Gerodontics* 1985;**1**:202–6.

Ocular prostheses

C STEVEN BAILEY, ROGER J BUCKLEY

Among people presenting to ophthalmology departments, the commonest requirements for cosmetic purposes are for whole eye prostheses that will disguise the absence of an eye and for various types of contact lens that will sit on the surface of a disfigured globe and act as a façade.

Whole eye prostheses

Indications for removing an eye include irreparable traumatic damage, malignancy, intractable suppuration, intractable pain in a blind eye, cosmetic reasons, and the prevention of sympathetic ophthalmitis. Removal may be by enucleation (when the whole eye is taken) or evisceration (when the contents of the scleral envelope are scooped out). Enucleation is always used for intraocular tumours and, usually, for pain. Evisceration is used when there may be a danger of intraocular infection spreading back along a cut optic nerve sheath. In other circumstances either operation can be used, although there is controversy over the merits and disadvantages of each.

At the end of the operation a simple conformer shell of clear Perspex must be inserted into the eye socket (fig 1) to prevent postoperative shrinkage of the orbital tissues, which would make it difficult to fit an artificial eye. Care must be exercised over cleanliness at this stage and at every other stage. As with all whole eye prostheses conformer shells should be removed for cleaning at least once every 24 hours.

Patients who have lost an eye are psychologically scarred, and the cosmetic deficit should be corrected at the earliest opportunity by fitting a temporary coloured prosthesis that has been modified from a stock shape. This can be done in a hospital eye department

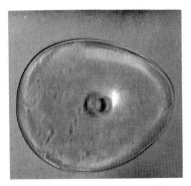

FIG 1—Simple conformer shell with vent for insertion after enucleation

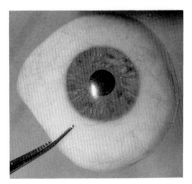

FIG 2—Whole eye prosthesis

that operates a prosthetic eye service or by the Artificial Eye Service. A final artificial eye can then be manufactured as soon as the postoperative inflammation has settled, commonly within six to 12 weeks. The device will usually be made in clinical quality Perspex, although glass may be used in selected cases.

To ensure that the eye sits in a natural position and does not fall back into the socket and to minimise any space in which infected debris could collect, the device should be shaped to match the contours of the orbital tissues. An impression of the socket is therefore taken using a quick setting material such as dental alginate. Once set, the alginate is removed and a plaster of Paris mould is made from it. The mould is used to cast a wax shape, which is then trimmed to fit the socket. A further mould is made from the modified wax shape, and the Perspex prosthesis is cast in this mould. A hand painted iris button is placed on the front of the eye, scleral features are painted on, and clear plastic is laminated over the top (fig 2).

Whole eye prostheses should be worn overnight during periods of orbital growth. They may continue to be worn overnight later, perhaps for the sake of a partner or else to prevent eyelashes turning in and irritating the conjunctival surface, but if conjunctival inflammation develops secondary to the device it is probably best not worn during sleep. To remove an artificial eye the edge of the lower eyelid is first manipulated under the inferior edge of the device. The superior aspect of the prosthesis is then pushed downwards by applying pressure to the upper lid skin crease.

Cleaning is best done by hand with a simple liquid surfactant such as baby shampoo. Liquid soaps should be avoided because they contain oils that will interfere with the wetting of the surface of the prosthesis. The surfactant must be rinsed off with water that has been boiled and cooled, and the shell can then be reinserted. It should not be dried: paper tissues will scratch the surface and towels are likely to be contaminated with microbes. After removal of the prosthesis the socket may be gently irrigated with sterile isotonic saline at body temperature. The saline is available from high street optical practices in single use sachets. A 20 ml hypodermic syringe is a suitable applicator.

Cosmetic contact lenses

Cosmetic contact lenses are intended to disguise eyes that have developed unacceptable appearances. They fall into three groups: scleral shells, soft corneoscleral contact lenses (hydrogel), and rigid corneal contact lenses (fig 3). Rigid lenses are unusual, and most patients will be fitted with one of the first two types.

Scleral shells

Scleral shells are indicated when the eye is shrunken or its surface is uneven. The thickness of the shell can be varied; a property that can be used to fill out the volume deficit that accompanies ocular atrophy. Attempts to fit such a device to a disfigured but normal sized eye may result in exophthalmos. Shells can hide a small degree of strabismus, but large angle squints in eyes with good ocular movements must be corrected surgically before a prosthesis is fitted. This is because the movement of the device will be limited unless unsightly gaps are left around it and if the eye behind it has a greater freedom of movement it will scrape across the posterior surface of the shell.

Scleral shells should be worn only while awake as the shell occludes the cornea, placing it under metabolic stress and increasing the risk of ulceration. The eye is anyway slightly stressed under the closed lid during sleep so it is advisable to remove the shell an hour or two before going to bed to encourage the corneal epithelium to recover. Because of the risk of ulceration more scrupulous care must be taken over the maintenance of a scleral shell than over a whole eye prosthesis. When the shell is removed in the evening it should be cleaned with a surfactant designed for rigid contact

100

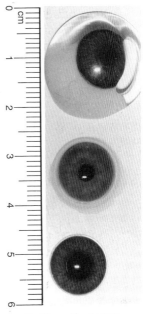

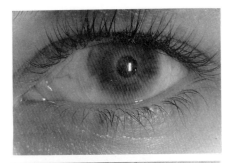

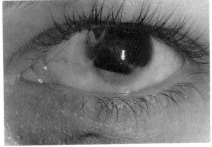

FIG 3—Cosmetic contact lenses (*from top to bottom*): scleral shell, soft corneoscleral lens, and Perspex lens

FIG 4—Eye with (*top*) and without (*bottom*) soft corneoscleral lens

lenses, rinsed in cool water that has been boiled, and put into a clean case filled with fresh rigid contact lens disinfecting solution. The necessary solutions are not available on NHS prescriptions, except when dispensed from a hospital pharmacy, but they can be readily obtained from high street optical practices.

Soft corneoscleral lenses

These lenses are used to hide corneal scars and iris defects in normal sized eyes that have a fairly regular surface (fig 4). Corneal scarring may occur after trauma or infection. Iris defects are usually induced by trauma but may be congenital. Soft lenses cannot be used if the eye is so misshaped that the lens will not centre or if the tear film is deficient. These lenses can be fully occlusive, with both pupil and iris coloured to match the fellow eye, or they can have a clear pupil if the eye is sighted. In the latter case the lens may also be powered to correct a refractive error.

Soft lenses of this type must be worn only during waking hours

101

for the same reasons that apply to scleral shells. They must be cleaned and disinfected on removal with solutions designed for soft contact lenses. No other medium than sterile saline from a single use sachet or pressurised canister (both available from optical practices) is appropriate for rinsing them. Soft lens disinfecting solutions containing chlorine or hydrogen peroxide should not be used with these lenses because the colours will eventually become bleached. Fitting cosmetic contact lenses is a specialist task that is usually managed from suitably equipped hospital eye departments.

Complications

The problems associated with wearing scleral shells and cosmetic contact lenses are the same as for other types of contact lenses, but two conditions are worthy of special mention.

Papillary conjunctivitis

Papillary conjunctivitis associated with foreign bodies is common in wearers of whole eye prostheses and shells and can cause great distress. It represents a cell mediated hypersensitivity reaction to components of the deposits which collect on the surface of the device. These potential allergens are rendered more effective by being rubbed against the upper tarsal conjunctiva during blinking. Patients complain of local irritation, due to the release of inflammatory mediators, and of sticky discharge, due to excess mucus secretion. The upper tarsal conjunctiva is characteristically hyperaemic, infiltrated, and oedematous and often shows massive papillary hyperplasia. The condition may be controlled by ensuring that the prosthesis is kept scrupulously clean and by reducing the wearing time, but if these measures are not sufficient topical drugs may be considered.

Sodium cromoglycate eye drops used four times daily can be helpful, but sometimes topical steroids are required. Drops are preferable to ointment for long term treatment because the smearing of the prosthesis tends to be cosmetically unacceptable. It is not usually necessary to remove the artificial eye before applying the treatment. Steroids are not without hazard, even in the case of blind or absent eyes. Although frank infection is a relatively uncommon cause of discharge from a socket fitted into a prosthesis, this possibility should be considered before commencing treatment. Clinicians should not be tempted to try to cover all possibilities by prescribing an antibiotic and steroid combination that contains an aminoglycoside because of the risk of a hypersensitivity reaction.

Over 40% of cases of infective conjunctivitis are caused by *Staphylococcus aureus*, *Haemophilus* spp are responsible for a further 20% and streptococci for another 14%. The remaining 26% are due to organisms such as *Acinetobacter calcoaceticus*, *Steptococcus viridans*, *Neisseria gonorrhoeae*, *Moraxella* spp, *Proteus* spp, *Klebsiella pneumoniae*, *Streptococcus pyogenes*, and *Serratia marcescens*. *Pseudomonas aeruginosa* has occasionally been isolated.

Treatment with first line topical antibiotics, such as chloramphenicol, may be commenced after swabs have been taken. The prosthesis should be removed before any drugs are administered. Ointment used four times daily is usually acceptable for short term treatment and may be more effective than two hourly drops because compliance is likely to be better.

In the rare case of sterile papillary conjunctivitis that is resistant to all other measures the patient may have to be refitted with a hand blown glass eye. Glass provides a better wetting surface than Perspex and is also less likely to collect deposits. On the downside, glass eyes quickly become etched by tears and, as they cannot be effectively polished, they have to be replaced frequently. The life of a glass eye can vary from only six months to two years, whereas a well cared for Perspex prosthesis will last for many years and is therefore most cost effective. Furthermore, manufacturing glass eyes is a rare skill in Britain, there being only one technician in full time practice.

Post-enucleation socket syndrome

The post-enucleation socket syndrome occurs when the lower eyelid is stretched downwards by the mass of a whole eye prosthesis (fig 5). As the prosthesis sinks lower the upper lid also begins to droop, and a deep hollow forms under the superior orbital rim.

Replacing the artificial eye with one of a new shape may help the appearance in the early stages, but surgery is often ultimately required. Surgery entails correcting the eyelid positions with fascial slings and part filling the empty socket by implanting an inert device beneath the superficial orbital tissues. A thin, lightweight shell can then be made to replace the previous prosthesis.

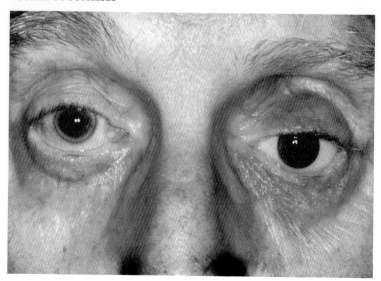

FIG 5—Post-enucleation socket syndrome in prosthetic left eye. Note upper and lower eyelid ptosis, deep upper palpebral sulcus, and appearance of enophthalmos

Appendix

A full range of cosmetic and prosthetic services are available from the Ocular Prosthetics Department, Manchester Royal Eye Hospital, Manchester M13 9WH (061 276 1234) and the Contact Lens and Prosthesis Department, Moorfields Eye Hospital, London EC1V 2PD (071 253 3411). Many other centres offer some facilities.

Details of local artificial eye service centres can be obtained from the main administrative unit at the Artificial Eye Service, Block 1, Room 103E, Government Buildings, Warbreck Hill Road, Blackpool FY2 0UZ.

Splints

PATRICIA M RILEY

A splint is a device applied to part of the body for protection or to help in restoring or improving function. Splints may be static or dynamic. Protective static splints prevent weak muscles being stretched and support joints by substituting for weak muscles. They are useful in cases of trauma and spinal cord injury and as resting splints for patients with rheumatoid arthritis. Corrective static splints force the affected joint into the correct or near correct alignment and are used for contracture of burn scars and tendon adhesions and as working splints for patients with rheumatoid arthritis. Dynamic splints give mobility to the patient's joints by providing forces that substitute for absent muscle power—for example, postoperative outriggers for metacarpophalangeal joint replacements.

Types of splint

Splints are either resting, working, or serial.

Resting splints maintain the joint in the optimum anatomical, rehabilitative, or prophylactic position. They work at night or during rest periods (in certain cases they may be used continually for a prescribed period). Night resting splints are commonly used to provide support and rest in the functional anatomical positions, but the splinted limb cannot be used functionally while the splint is in place. They are used in cases of rheumatoid arthritis, trauma, hand surgery, cerebrovascular accidents, burns, and skin grafts. Night resting splints are usually made in Orthoplast or Sansplint thermoplastic material (fig 1).

Working splints allow the patient to use the limb functionally while it is splinted. They usually hold one joint in a static position while other joints are free to function—for example, wrist splints

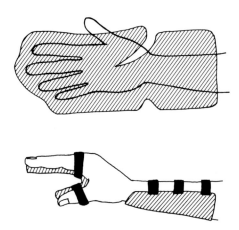

FIG 1—Night resting splint. *Top*: pattern; *bottom*: in position with velcro straps

allow full elbow and finger movement. They may incorporate a dynamic component, giving assisted or resisted movement. Wrist working splints are commonly used in cases of rheumatoid arthritis to ease and protect painful wrist joints, thus ensuring a more stable wrist to carry out functional activity. These splints are also used in cases of the carpal tunnel syndrome, as maintaining the wrist in an extended position eases symptoms, and in cases of trauma. They are usually made from Plastazote and Vitrathene, providing a flexible yet supportive splint and allow full movement of the metacarpophalangeal joint (fig 2).

High profile dynamic outriggers (fig 3) may be used in metacarpophalangeal joint replacement and trauma. They allow flexion of the joints but maintain them in extension. They may be used as part of a postoperative regimen for a specified time.

Serial splints may be resting or working splints. They are used to improve gradually the range of movement by regular readjustment of the splint to stretch soft tissue or joint contracture.

The ideal splint must be neat, comfortable, lightweight, durable, washable, individually and simply designed, free of pressure areas (unless pressure is required in specific cases such as in patients with burn scars), easily adjustable, and understood by the patient, staff, and relatives concerned.

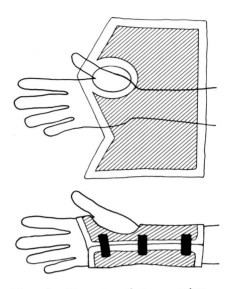

FIG 2—Wrist working splint. *Top*: pattern; *bottom*: complete

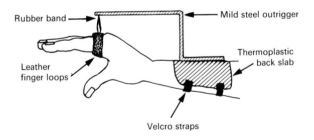

FIG 3—High profile dynamic outrigger

Who needs a splint?

There are several conditions in which splints can help in rehabilitating and managing patients.

Rheumatoid arthritis—In this condition splints can be used as part of a joint protection programme to keep them in alignment, ease pain, and rest them in a functional position. Splints do not prevent ulnar drift or permanently correct it but may slow down the process if used with joint protection techniques. Splints that temporarily provide joint alignment enable the patient to have better function.

Burn scars—Where there is burned tissue it is important that the joints are maintained in the optimum anatomical position. This helps to maintain function and prevent contracture. If contractures have formed in immature scar tissue serial splinting is possible to gradually stetch out the scar.

Flexor tendon injuries—Postoperatively surgeons commonly request dynamic splinting to a repaired tendon to allow movement through the tendon sheath while not exerting any force of movement on it. Once the tendon has healed serial splinting may be required to stretch the tendon and help release adhesions.

Neurological conditions that result in poor function—for example, motor neurone disease and tetraplegia due to either traumatic spinal cord injury or other means—may benefit from resting splints that maintain the optimum position of function and working splints that provide increased means of function. Certain conditions that result in spasticity of a limb may benefit from splinting. Splinting the palmar surface of a spastic hand, however, may increase the tone and thereby worsen the condition. A variety of other types of splints not applied to the palmar surface may be used. Even when it is a longstanding problem (older than six months) palmar splinting may not be contraindicated and can actively help to improve function and reduce pain.

Trauma resulting from crush injuries and fractures often requires support in a functional position in the form of resting, working, or serial splints.

Who provides splints?

Splints are usually provided by hospital based occupational therapists, who learn the techniques of splint making as part of their training. Orthotists may also be involved through a hospital's surgical appliance department. They are usually apprentice trained by commercial companies that provide surgical appliances and visit hospitals on a sessional basis.

What materials are used?

Thermoplastic materials are used as they can be softened and moulded with either dry or wet heat to the appropriate style and position. Orthotists usually use high temperature materials, which can only be shaped on a mould and not directly on to the patient's limb. Occupational therapists use low temperature materials, which can be moulded directly on to the patient. The use of low temperature materials means that the splint may be made with relative ease and speed. The patient can be assessed and fitted and leave hospital with the splint in place often in one or two hours. As there are changes in the patient's condition the splint may be easily adjusted as required. Some commonly used materials are Orthoplast, Sansplint, Hexcelite, Plastazote, and Orfit.

How can splinting be successful?

The initial prescription for splinting must be appropriate and the doctor responsible for the patient needs to discuss what is required with the therapists concerned and a plan of the treatment needs to be organised. The therapist and doctor must have good lines of communication and be aware of the use and limitations of splinting. Follow up must be regular, by both the doctor and the therapist, and progress charted. The patient and the carer (if appropriate) need explanations of the splinting regimen so that they can participate in it and be motivated to use the splint. Finally, it is essential to remember that a splint is only part of the total treatment received by the patient yet has equal importance to those other treatments.

Appendix

Recommended reading

Turner A. *The practice of occupational therapy*. Edinburgh: Livingstone, 1981.

Moberg E. *Splinting in hand therapy*. New York: Thieme Stratton, 1984.

Malik M. *Manual of static hand splinting*. Pittsburg, Pennsylvania: Harmaville Rehabilitation Centre, 1976.

Malik M. *Manual of dynamic hand splinting*. Pittsburgh, Pennsylvania: Harmaville Rehabilitation Centre, 1976.

Zislis JM. Splinting of the hand in a spastic hemiplegic patient. *Arch Phys Med Rehabil* 1964;**45**:41–3.

Snook JH. Spasticity reduction splint. *Am J Occup Ther* 1979;**33**:648–50.

Ellis M. Splinting the rheumatoid hand. *Clinics in Rheumatic Diseases* 1984;**10**:673–95.

Clarke C, Allard L, Braybrooks B. *Rehabilitation in rheumatology*. London: Dunitz, 1987.

Goodwill CJ, Chamberlain MA. *Rehabilitation of the physically disabled adult*. London: Croom Helm, 1988.

Trusses

E BURNS, A WHITLEY

A hernia is the protrusion of a viscus or a part of a viscus through an abnormal opening in the walls of its containing cavity. The commonest forms of external abdominal hernias are inguinal, femoral, and umbilical.

All hernias are at risk of strangulation or obstruction, and although the risk of these complications may vary with the site and nature of the hernia (table), even an easily reducible direct inguinal defect is not without risk. Therefore the best treatment for any hernia is surgery. Surgery should always be considered for femoral hernias: not only is the risk of strangulation high but a truss is rarely effective in maintaining reduction of the hernia as the hernial sac protrudes into the leg and movement of the leg results in descent of the hernial contents.[1] The hazards of emergency treatment of a strangulated or obstructed hernia exceed considerably those of elective surgical repair and therefore patients should be advised to opt for operative treatment, especially as surgery may be performed under spinal or even local anaesthesia if the patient's condition precludes general anaesthesia.[2]

External abdominal hernias: prevalence of relative risks of strangulation or obstruction

Site of hernia	Prevalence (%)*	Estimated risk of complication
Inguinal:		
Indirect	10·0	High
Direct	63·0	Moderate
Femoral	17·0	Very high
Umbilical	8·5	Variable but usually moderate

*Excluding epigastric, paraumbilical, spigelian, lumbar, gluteal, and sciatic hernias (comprising in total the remaining 1·5% of external abdominal hernias).

A truss may be considered for patients who are too frail for or who refuse surgery and for patients awaiting operation. The aims of treatment are to prevent strangulation or obstruction of the hernia and to reduce the local discomfort of the defect.

Are trusses useful?

Few studies of the efficacy and acceptability of trusses have been reported. To maintain reduction of a hernia the pressure produced by the truss must be directed along the line of descent of the hernia. As the hernial canal passes obliquely through the abdominal wall the force produced by the truss must be directed upwards and backwards. This aim is rarely achieved, so that protrusion of the hernial contents into the canal is not prevented by the truss even if descent into the hernial sac does not occur. Therefore the risk of strangulation or obstruction is likely to remain,[3 4] but trusses usually relieve the symptoms.

One study reported on 85 patients who were treated before operation with a truss for periods ranging from one month to 42 years.[5] This was a retrospective review with no untreated controls, and the subjects had all been selected for treatment with elective surgery. Almost all of the patients used an elastic truss. Almost a third (24 patients) experienced complete relief from hernial discomfort and a further third (29) reported some improvement in their symptoms. The remaining 26% (22 patients) had a variety of difficulties: the discomfort of the truss exceeded that of the hernia itself in nine; the hernia became incarcerated in six; one patient suffered ipsilateral testicular atrophy, and in the remaining seven the truss was considered "ineffective." No prospective controlled studies of the use of trusses have been reported.

Problems with trusses

Some of the problems encountered with a truss have been described above. The use of a truss may itself increase the risk of hernial complications. Pressure on the margins of the hernial orifice may lead to atrophy of the fascia and aponeurosis, enlarging the hernial defect, and longstanding use of a truss may result in adhesion of the spermatic cord to the hernial sac—both these problems tend to make surgical repair more difficult. Pressure on a protruding hernial mass from a truss may impair venous and lymphatic return and increase the risk of strangulation. Other complications of the use of a truss are atrophy of the spermatic cord, the development of adhesions within the hernial sac, and thrombosis of the iliac artery.[3]

Types of truss

Two types of truss are commonly prescribed: the elastic and spring truss (fig 1). The two types vary in the composition of the belt of the truss, but the design has changed little since James Parkinson offered his "hints for the improvement of the truss" in 1802.[6] The most common construction is a belt either of elastic webbing or of a spring covered in cotton or linen, with a pad designed to hold the hernia in reduction attached to the belt. A "rat tail" strap forms a perineal support, holding the pad against the hernial orifice (fig 2). The pad and the anterior portion of the strap are covered with cotton or linen, and the posterior section of the perineal strap is constructed of elastic webbing. Maintaining the truss is difficult as none of its components are removable or washable. Trusses may be supplied as single or double as requird for unilateral or bilateral deficits.

Frail patients may have difficulty in manipulating a spring truss as considerable strength may be required to fit it, and many patients find such trusses too uncomfortable to wear. The elastic truss is usually better tolerated, although fitting of even this design requires a degree of manual dexterity as the elastic belt must first be fastened tightly and the perineal strap then secured by fastening a buckle at the back of the elastic belt.

Large irreducible hernias may provoke considerable discomfort. If surgery is impossible symptoms may be relieved by supporting the hernial contents with a bag truss (fig 3).

Prescribing

A truss may be prescribed on the standard form (FP10) by either general practitioners or hospital doctors. It is important that the patient is directed to a qualified surgical appliance supplier (an orthotist) so that the support may be correctly fitted; if necessary the orthotist may arrange for alteration of the truss. The orthotist will also instruct the patient in fitting the truss.

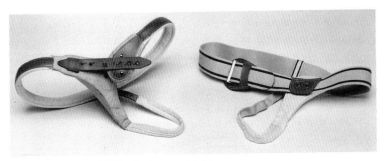

FIG 1—Spring truss (*left*); elastic truss (*right*)

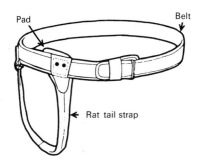

FIG 2—Truss showing belt, pad, and rat tail strap

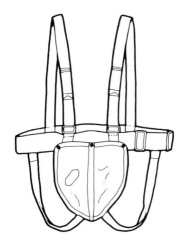

FIG 3—Bag truss

Practical hints to patients

Information to patients on fitting and maintaining their truss is based on common sense rather than the results of scientific endeavour. The patient must always be recumbent and the hernia fully reduced when the truss is fitted. If the appliance is uncomfortable the orthotists can arrange for suitable alteration; they are also the best source of further advice to the patient. In most cases, however, orthotists rarely see the patient after supplying the truss. If a replacement is required a new prescription should be issued.

We thank Mr PJ Finan for helpful criticism of the manuscript.

1 Rains RDH, Ritchie HD. *Bailey and Love's short practice of surgery.* 20th ed. London: HK Lewis, 1988.
2 Condon RF, Nyhus LM. Complications of groin hernia repair. *Surg Clin N Am* 1971;**51**:1325–36.
3 Scher AD, Bolton NJ. Iliac artery thrombosis associated with the use of a truss. *Arch Surg* 1969;**98**:758–9.
4 Harris FI, White AS. The truss in relationship to diagnosis and injection of inguinal hernia. *Am J Surg* 1937;**36**:443–61.
5 Ljungdahl I. Inguinal and femoral hernia. *Acta Chir Scand* 1973;suppl 439:7–77.
6 Parkinson J. *Hints for the improvement of trusses; intended to render their use less inconvenient, and to prevent the necessity of an understrap. With the description of a truss of easy construction and slight expense, for the use of a labouring poor to whom this little tract is chiefly addressed.* London: HD Symonds, 1802.

Wigs

M J CHEESBROUGH

Wigs were originally popularised in Britain by Queen Elizabeth I, who is said to have owned no fewer than 80, and Mary Queen of Scots is reputed to have worn one at her execution. Louis XIII of France went prematurely bald in 1624 and by disguising his baldness with a wig started a fashion that lasted over 150 years. In the seventeenth century the grandest wigs were worn by the wealthy and important, hence the expression "big wigs." The demand for wigs was so great that children were forbidden to go out alone in case thieves cut off their hair.

Today five types of wig are worn: necessity wigs to cover baldness, fashion or fun wigs, legal wigs, wigs worn for religious reasons, and theatrical wigs. Necessity and fun wigs merely differ in their indications for use. A variety of fibres are used in their construction, but the commonest material is acrylic, which makes high quality and fairly cheap wigs.

Significance of hair

The large number of salons in every high street bears witness to the importance of the state and style of the hair to people's self image. Few people are unconcerned by losing hair, and for many alopecia is deeply upsetting. There are no objective studies of the psychological effects of alopecia, but Elizabeth Steel in her book *Coping with Sudden Hair Loss* describes the effects it had on her.[1] Through case histories she highlights a common thread of shock, unhappiness, loss of confidence, and work, social, and sexual difficulties combined with feelings of lack of understanding by health professionals. Furthermore, patients with disorders of self image (dysmorphophobia) often have symptoms referable to their

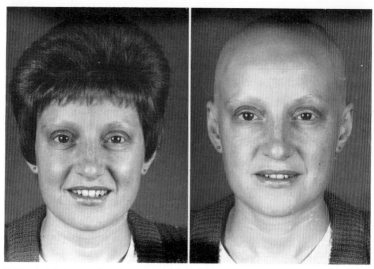

Patient with severe alopecia areata with and without her wig

hair or scalp,[2] which suggests a deep seated psychological importance of the head and scalp as well as other anatomical sites.

The Department of Health recognises the distress that alopecia
causes and therefore allows wigs to be prescribed through the
NHS. These can be prescribed only by hospital consultants, and
most are prescribed by dermatologists, neurosurgeons, radiothera-
pists, and oncologists. Although wigs can be supplied for men,
women, and children, 70 of the 74 patients provided with wigs by
Huddersfield Health Authority in 1987–8 were women. An
unknown number buy their wigs privately.

Criteria for supply of wigs

The Department of Health's regulations state that wigs may be
provided only when a consultant considers one to be necessary and
when the baldness is due to any of the following conditions: (*a*)
congenital dystrophy of the skin; (*b*) alopecia totalis; (*c*) alopecia
areata (severe and long standing); (*d*) extensive scarring after
trauma, *x* ray application, or an inflammatory condition; (*e*) illness
or treatment when baldness, though not permanent, is likely to be
prolonged (for example, after intracranial operation or radiotherapy); and (*f*) prolonged administration of cytotoxic drugs.

As the regulations state that "it is not the intention that normal male baldness should itself justify the provision of a wig under the National Health Service, nor that elderly (*ie* over the age of 70) female patients whose hair is thinning due to normal aging, qualify ..." (*National Health Service Provision of Medical and Surgical Appliances*, paras 23 and 24) baldness due to physiological hair loss is therefore excluded. In a dermatologist's practice most patients' baldness is due to alopecia areata or totalis—that is, alopecia areata affecting the whole of the scalp. I prescribe wigs for anyone who wants one providing he or she fulfils the regulations.

Construction of wigs

The base or foundation is made first and is either hard or soft. Hard bases are made from flexible plastic or fibreglass and soft bases from cotton, terylene or nylon, or silk and may be partly or completely lined. Hard bases are never used for real hair wigs and are mainly found in men's wigs to provide better adhesion. The hair may be either real or acrylic. Acrylic is now so good that few real hair wigs are prescribed on the NHS (though consultants have to specify which they require for the patient). Real hair wigs are usually made from European human hair, but hair from Asians or animal hair (such as yak hair) may be used. Acrylic wigs are cheaper and easier to care for and clean. They can be hand washed by their owners whereas real hair wigs have to be dry cleaned by a specialist.

Supply of wigs

The normal route for supply of wigs on the NHS is for the consultant to send the patient, with the prescription, to the appliance officer, who organises the administrative and financial details. The patient is then passed on to the hospital "wig agent," who is normally a trained hairdresser and attends the hospital regularly. The agent helps the patient to choose the appropriate style and colour, and the available choice is extremely wide. Real hair wigs have to be made to measure and the agent takes the necessary measurements, whereas acrylic wigs are stock sizes and adjusted to any head. Samples and colour brochures are available to help the patients make a choice, and when indicated the agent may make a domiciliary visit at the hospital's expense. When the wig has been chosen an order is placed with a regional health authority contractor, and after delivery the agent is responsible for checking its fitting and instructing the patient in its care and maintenance. Acrylic wigs are usually delivered within a few days, but real hair wigs may take eight to 12 weeks.

Whether patients get their wigs from hospital or outside it is important that private fitting rooms are available; bald patients have complained of their embarrassment at having to try on wigs in the concourse of department stores or hospital appliance departments.

Renewal and costs

Patients are usually supplied with two wigs (one to wear and one to clean). In this hospital acrylic wigs are replaced at the rate of one a year and human hair wigs at the rate of two every three years, but there are no official rules and consultants have discretion. Patients vary in the rate at which their wig wears out, and it is not necessary for consultants to see patients for each renewal; they can give a long term prescription for as long as they want.

At present, patients pay £26 for each acrylic wig and £97 for each real hair wig, which represents about two thirds the real cost of them. National figures for total expenditure on wigs by the NHS are not kept, but Huddersfield Health Authority supplied 104 wigs to 74 patients in 1987–8 at a total expenditure of about £3700. The estimated national expenditure by the 200 health districts would therefore be about £740 000, which is about three quarters of the expenditure on drugs for a single district.

Patients who are in hospital when their wigs are supplied are entitled to free wigs, as are outpatients under the age of 16, 16 to 19 year olds still in full time education, and patients receiving income support or family credit. People on low incomes may be entitled to help with the cost of wigs, and the precise criteria are described in leaflet WF11/April 1988, which can be found in any hospital or Department of Health office.

Care of wigs

All wigs should be dry combed and brushed daily like normal hair, but they must not be combed or brushed when wet. If the wig does get wet in the rain or when the wearer is swimming it should

Do's and Don't's

Acrylic wigs

1 Wash in luke warm water with a cold rinse
2 Do not use a hair dryer. Heat damages acrylic fibres and can make them frizzle or melt, but they do not catch fire
3 Keep away from direct heat
4 Do not apply heated rollers but cold rollers can be used

Human hair wigs

1 Avoid soaking in water as this loosens the hand knotting. It may also cause matting of the hair
2 Dry clean by specialist only. This is arranged by the appliance officer and patients are allowed one free clean a month (cost to the NHS £6)
3 Heated rollers can be used
4 Only have the wig permed professionally because of the risk of damage from water
5 Do not dye the hair unless it is done professionally

be allowed to dry before combing or it will matt. Decorations such as ribbons, butterfly combs, and hats can be worn. The agent will normally give further advice on looking after wigs and can be contacted directly or through the appliance officer. The box gives a list of do's and don't's for the care of wigs.

Wig blocks can be used for storage, but wigs can be folded and put away in a drawer when not in use. An adjustable strap is provided at the back of acrylic wigs and for women this is all that is required to keep the wig in place. Optional two sided adhesive pads can be used for extra security in women and these are essential for male toupees (partial wigs or hairpieces to cover incomplete baldness). Some men find better adhesion with wigs with hard rather than soft bases. Being bespoke, real hair wigs should stay in place without any extra help.

Complications and acceptability

Irritation and allergy from the materials can occur but are exceptionally rare and have never happened in any of my patients. Were this to occur the offending material would have to be identified by patch testing so that a wig free of the substance could be made.

Patients make few complaints about the wigs supplied and the fact that most continue to wear them out and come back for replacements attests to their cosmetic acceptability. You should explain to patients that they are not getting NHS wigs but that the NHS is making a financial contribution to the provision of a fashionable wig, which should at least bring the patient back to his or her former appearance and may even enhance it. A *Which?* report on male hair pieces in 1969 questioned users on the pros and cons of wigs.[3] Respondents felt that the advantages of hair pieces included looking younger, increased confidence, warming of the head, and protection from knocks. The disadvantages reported included the feeling of being committed to wearing a wig to maintain the secrecy of baldness, a tendency for the colour to change or fade, being uncomfortably hot in summer, disarrangement by wind, needing more care than natural hair, and the possibility of looking younger than one's wife.

1 Steel E. *Coping with sudden hair loss.* Wellingborough, Northamptonshire: Thorsons Publishing Group, 1988.
2 Cotterill JA. Dermatological non-disease: a common and potentially fatal disturbance of body image. *Br J Dermatol* 1981;**104**:611.
3 Consumers Association. Hairpieces for men. *Which?* 1969 October:313–9.

Appendix

Helpful information

Leaflet WF11/April 1988 from hospitals, Department of Health offices or leaflets unit, Box 21, Stanmore, Middlesex, HA7 1AY.
Hairline International, Chantry Vellacott, Chartered Accountants, Post and Mail House, Colmore Circus, Birmingham, B4 6AT (please enclose stamped addressed envelope). This is a self help organisation.

Further reading

Woodforde J. *The strange story of false hair.* London: Routledge and Kegan Paul, 1971.
Consumers Association. Wigs and hairpieces for women. *Which?* 1971 Feb:49–55.

Mobility aids

Aids for disabled drivers

CHRISTIAN MURRAY-LESLIE

Disabled people may require driving aids to enable them to drive for the first time, to adjust to increasing disability (as with progressive disorders such as rheumatoid arthritis and multiple sclerosis), or to return to driving after a single disabling illness (such as a stroke, amputation, or injury to the spinal cord).

Assessment and advice—The disabled person should first obtain medical advice from his or her general practitioner or medical specialist. When applying for a driving licence for the first time the applicant will be asked questions on disabling conditions. If a person already has a driving licence and has subsequently developed a disability that might affect driving safety he or she is obliged by law to notify the medical branch of the Driver and Vehicle Licensing Centre at Swansea as soon as possible. If there is no bar to driving but there is uncertainty about the feasibility or safety of driving advice may be sought from any one of the 10 United Kingdom driving assessment centres (see appendix). The centres provide impartial and non-commercial advice based on the assessment of driving capabilities and need for aids. Assessments on a static test module are usually followed by a test drive in a suitably adapted vehicle on a private road.

Choice of vehicle—When choosing a motor vehicle a disabled person and his or her advisers need to consider several points: (*a*) How will I and my passenger (who may also be disabled) get in and out of the car? (*b*) Are there problems of wheelchair access and stowage? (*c*) Would I like to drive from a wheelchair? (*d*) Is an automatic transmission necessary or desirable? (*e*) Is power assisted steering necessary or desirable?

Access—Cars with two rather than four side doors generally provide a much wider aperture and therefore better access for both the driver and front seat passenger. Some manufacturers supply a disabled driver's model of a standard two door saloon, which includes extended seat runners to allow greater retraction of the front seat. Extended seat runners can be fitted to most cars from upwards of £40, depending upon the vehicle model. Advice on getting in and out of cars, including wheelchair transfers, hoisting, and stowage, is given in an excellent booklet published by the Department of Transport.

Driving from a wheelchair is achieved in two ways. Firstly, the disabled person in his or her wheelchair is hoisted into the empty seat well of the car, or, secondly, a specially adapted vehicle is used and the wheelchair and its occupant enters by a ramp at the rear or side of the vehicle, the seating having been removed. Secure anchorage of the wheelchair and the wearing of a seat belt securely attached to the vehicle frame to the test standards of the Department of Transport is essential.

Automatic or manual transmission—Some disabled drivers—for example, those with hemiplegia or those without any use in their legs, such as paraplegics—will require vehicles with automatic transmission, and others—for example, those with painful arthritic joints—may also benefit. Fortunately, many smaller vehicles now have automatic gearboxes. Currently 45 models of car under 1·6 l engine size are available with automatic transmission.

Power assisted steering may be essential to people with neurological impairment of their arms and of considerable help to those with painful conditions of the arms and spine.

Swivel seats (fig 1)—Access to vehicles can be improved by converting the existing car seat so that it is capable of rotating in and out of the car or by removing the existing seat and installing a special swivel seat. The price of these seats and the cost of fitting ranges from about £175 to £335. The seat should be capable of being locked in the rotated out position and have a headrest. Ideally it should be capable of sliding backwards and forwards in addition to rotating and have a good seat back, which can be reclined. "Leather look" seats that have less friction will help transfers in and out of a wheelchair.

Seat cushions—Many disabled people will drive sitting on a cushion for comfort, to prevent pressure sores, or because they are short in stature. If cushions are used with the usual lap and

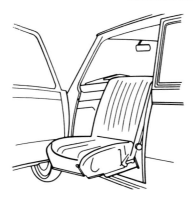

FIG 1—Swivel seat. (Reproduced from *Ins and Outs of Car Choice* by kind permission of the Department of Transport)

diagonally fitted seat belts they should be firmly constructed and anchored to the back of the seat. If the cushions are soft or filled with air they should be enclosed in a firm cover and firmly anchored to the back of the seat to prevent abdominal injuries from seat belts.

Seat belts—Disabled drivers and disabled passengers should generally wear seat belts and certificates of permanent exemption from use are seldom justified. Some people, however, do have problems with seat belts. Some prefer the static rather than the inertia belts. If an inertia belt is used one with a lower recoil force may be more comfortable to wear and easier to fasten. Comfort clips to reduce tension in an inertia system by including slack in the belt can reduce their safety and must be fitted carefully. Lowering the upper anchorage point of the belt may reduce pressure on the side of the neck. Disabled people commonly experience difficulty in reaching seat belts, and this can be cheaply and safely achieved by using a simple clip on extension handle (fig 2). The difficulty disabled people experience in fastening and unfastening seat belts can be remedied by using a different system, such as a static or inertia belt with less recoil, or a buckle.

Car keys (fig 3)—People with weak or arthritic hands may have difficulty manipulating the key either in the car door or in the ignition switch. Most occupational therapy departments or re-habilitation workshops can make simple modifications to the base of the key to help grip.

125

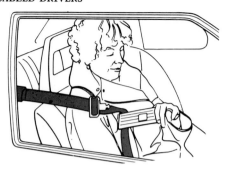

FIG 2—Clip on seat belt extension handle. (Reproduced from *Ins and Outs of Car Choice* by kind permission of the Department of Transport)

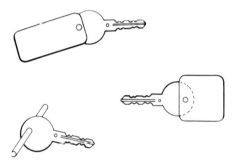

FIG 3—Car key handle modifications to assist gripping. (Reproduced from *Ins and Outs of Car Choice* by kind permission of the Department of Transport)

Additional car mirrors—Some drivers with severely restricted neck movement (such as in advanced ankylosing spondylitis or severe cervical spondylosis) may not be able to see to the rear with standard car mirrors. They must report their disability to the licensing authority. Panoramic mirrors, which can be clipped on to the interior driving mirror, give an increased field of vision to the rear of the vehicle. Difficulties with reverse parking in those with restricted neck mobility can be helped by using an angled lens fitted to the rear window, in conjunction with a standard interior rear view mirror.

Steering knob (fig 4)—Those who need to steer with one hand will require a knob to be attached to the steering wheel, which will allow adequate grip from full wheel lock to full wheel lock. People using a steering knob will include paraplegics who require the

126

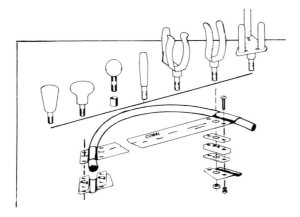

FIG 4—Variety of steering knobs and spinners with cross wheel brace

other hand to operate the brake and accelerator and those with hemiplegia who can use one foot for the brake and accelerator but who have only one functional hand with which to steer. People with weak or absent grip in both hands will require a specialised tetraplegic steering spinner. Such spinners are available in different shapes and sizes. Conventionally, steering knobs are positioned at the 10 o'clock and 2 o'clock positions for left and right handed use respectively. Some drivers, however, find other positions more comfortable. The effective use of a steering knob can be supplemented by using a vehicle with light steering or by ultralight power assisted steering.

Hand controls—A hand operated accelerator and brake are necessary when a driver does not have the use of both legs. These controls are generally used with an automatic gearbox, the driver steering with the other hand (usually the left) by using a wheel mounted steering knob. Design of hand controls varies, but the system usually works on an extended lever system attached to the conventional accelerator and brake pedals and mounted by the steering column (fig 5). Acceleration is achieved by pulling the handle towards the driver and braking by pushing the lever away. The systems are inexpensive (on average about £150), and there are several specialist conversion firms who will undertake the work (see appendix). When driving a vehicle fitted with hand controls the driver may take the other hand off the steering wheel when the vehicle is stationary to engage or disengage the handbrake.

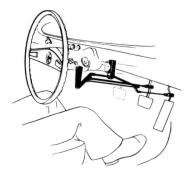

FIG 5—Accelerator and brake operated by right hand

Left accelerator conversions (fig 6)—For people who have had their right leg amputated any higher than the ankle and patients who have suffered a right hemiparesis a left sided accelerator will be needed with the brake pedal in its usual position.

Hand brake aids (fig 7) lengthen the hand brake to help the person with a short reach and make the handle of the brake easier to grip and the inhibitor button easier to release. These adaptations are useful to any person with weak painful hands. Again these aids are fairly cheap and can be obtained and fitted by car conversion specialists.

Costs—Providing aids will entail some extra expense, often fairly small and less than £200, but a change of vehicle would be more expensive. Much more expensive, sophisticated systems include

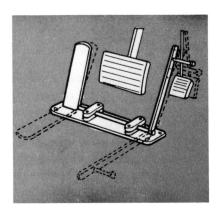

FIG 6—Flip up–flip down left accelerator conversion

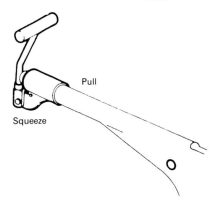

Pull

Squeeze

FIG 7—Hand brake release aid

remote joystick steering or specialised vehicles or adaptations to enable the person to drive from a wheelchair. Mobility allowance and its associated concessions, such as exemption from vehicle excise duty (car tax) and the conversion of mobility allowance to vehicle purchase or hire by instalments through the motability scheme, may do much to defray costs (see appendix). Unfortunately, mobility allowance is not available to those who have disabilities of the arms alone and who may require driving aids and, though paid until the age of 80, must be applied for before the 65th birthday.

Appendix

Driving assessment centres

Banstead Mobility Centre, Damson Way, Orchard Hill, Queen Mary's Avenue, Carshalton, Surrey SM5 4MR (081 770 1151).*
Derby Disabled Driving Centre, Kingsway Hospital, Kingsway, Derby DE3 3LZ (0332 371929).*
Mobility Advice and Vehicle Information Service, Department of Transport, TRRL, Crowthorne, Berkshire RG11 6AU (0344 770456. Information service only 071 212 5257).
Mobility Centre, Hunter's Moor Hospital, Newcastle upon Tyne NE2 4NR (091 2610895).
Mobility Information Service, Unit 2A, Atcham Estate, Upton Magna, Shrewsbury SY6 6UG (0743 75889).
Northern Ireland Council on Disability, 2 Annadale Avenue, Belfast BT7 3JR (0232 640011).

Rookwood Driving Assessment Centre, Rookwood Hospital, Llandaff, Cardiff CF5 2YN (0222 566281).

Stoke Mandeville Hospital, Occupational Therapy Workshop, Mandeville Road, Aylesbury, Buckinghamshire HP21 8AL (0296 84111).

Tehidy Friends Mobility Centre, Tehidy, Camborne, Cornwall TR14 0SA (0209 710708).*

The Mobility Centre, Hunter's Moor Hospital, Hunter's Road, Newcastle upon Tyne NE2 4NR (091 210454).

Vehicles for the Disabled Centre, Astley Ainslie Hospital, 133 Grange Loan, Edinburgh EH9 2HL (031 667 3398).*

Wales Disabled Drivers' Assessment Centre, 18 Plas Newydd, Whitchurch, Cardiff (0222 615276).

Centres that also provide medical assessments.

Car modification firms

London area

Automobile and Industrial Developments Ltd, Queensdale Works, Queensthorpe Road, Sydenham, London SE26 4JP (081 778 7055).

Feeny and Johnson (Components) Ltd, Alperton Lane, Wembley, Middlesex HA0 1JJ (081 998 4458).

D G Hodge and Son Ltd, Feathers Lane, Wraysbury, Staines, Middlesex (078481 3580).

Reselco Engineering Ltd, Kew Bridge Pumping Station, Green Dragon Lane, Brentford, Middlesex TW8 0EF (081 847 4509).

South

Wards Mobility Services Ltd, Ware Works, Bells Yew Lane, Tunbridge Wells, Kent TN3 9BD (089275 686).

Poynting Conversions, Faraday Road, Churchfields Industrial Estate, Salisbury, Wiltshire SP2 7NR (0722 33 6048).

Cowal (Mobility Aids) Ltd, 32 Newpond Road, Holmer Green, Near High Wycombe, Buckinghamshire HP15 6SU (044 714400).

Brig-Ayd Controls, Warrengate, Tewin, Welwyn, Hertfordshire AL6 0JD (043871 4206).

Brian Page, Specialist Auto Mechanics, 18 Pooley Green Road, Egham, Surrey TW20 8AF (0784 35850).

Steering Developments Ltd, Unit 3, Eastman Way, Hemel Hempstead, Hertfordshire HP2 7HF (0442 212918).

Interbility Ltd, 5 Badminton Close, Bragbury End, Stevenage, Hertfordshire SG2 8SR (0438 813365).

South west

Adaptacar, Cooks Cross, South Molton, North Devon EX36 4AW (07695 2785).

Philip Willey, Box 19, Portishead, Bristol BS20 8AS (0272 845061).

Midlands

Ashley Mobility, Hay Road, Hay Mills, Birmingham B25 8HY (021 772 5364).

Derby Disabled Driving Centre, Kingsway Hospital, Kingsway, Derby DE3 3LZ (0332 371929).

Midland Cylinder Rebores Ltd, Torrington Avenue, Coventry, West Midlands CV4 9BL (0203 462424).

Ross Auto Engineering Ltd, 2/3 Westfield Road, Wallasey, Cheshire L44 7HX (051 653 6000).

North

Alfred Bekker, The Green, Langtoft, Near Driffield, North Humberside YO25 0TF (0377 87276).

Eurostag (Leeds) Ltd, Wellbridge Industrial Estate, Wellington Bridge, Leeds 12 (0532 444765).

Motor Services (Manchester) Ltd, Royal Works, Canal Side, Edge Lane, Stretford, Near Manchester M32 8HS (061 865 6922).

SWS Motor Bodies, Unit 9, Hartford House, Newport Road, Weston Street, Bolton, Lancashire (0204 395660).

KC Mobility Services, Unit 4A, Victoria Mills, Bradford Road, Batley, West Yorkshire WF17 8LN (0924 442386).

Mobility allowance

A non-taxable, non-contributory benefit paid monthly to severely disabled people aged over 5.

To be eligible an applicant must: (*a*) be unable to walk or virtually unable to walk; (*b*) apply before 65th birthday; and (*c*) be able to make use of the allowance (for example, not be in a coma).

It may be spent on any form of mobility assistance.

It enables a person to hold a driving licence from the age of 16.

It entitles a person to possess an orange badge for privileged parking.

It gives exemption from vehicle excise licence duty (road tax).

It enables a person to use the motability scheme.

Motability scheme

Motability is a voluntary organisation set up by government initiative to help disabled people use their mobility allowance in instalment payments to obtain a car or electric wheel chair. Hire purchase and hiring agreements are made with Motability Finance Ltd, a special company that negotiates favourable financial terms with motor manufacturers, banks, etc. When an agreement is entered into the entire mobility allowance must be paid over for the duration of the agreement (four and a half years for vehicle purchase, three years for vehicle hire). A list of cars available for purchase and hire and the cost is available from Motability. When a vehicle is hired the cost of servicing and repairs are included in the rental, but when a vehicle is being purchased the user must pay for the repairs and maintenance.

Further details are available from Motability, Gate House, West Gate, The High, Harlow, Essex CM20 1HR (0279 635666).

Further information and recommended reading

The ins and outs of car choice. London: Department of Transport and Institute of Consumer Ergonomics, 1985.

Cochrane GM, Wiltshire ER, eds. *Outdoor transport.* 6th ed. Oxford: Mary Marlborough Lodge, 1987. (Equipment for Disabled series.)

Royal Commission on Accident Prevention In: Raffle A, ed. *Medical aspects of fitness to drive.* London: HMSO, 1985.

Darnborough A, Kinrade D. *Motoring and mobility for disabled people.* 4th ed. London: Royal Association for Rehabilitation and Disability, 1988.

Motability leaflet prepared by Motability, Gate House, West Gate, The High, Harlow, Essex CM20 1HR.

Mobility Allowance. (Leaflet NI 211.) DSS Mobility Allowance Unit, Norcross, Blackpool FY5 3TA (0253 856123).

Callipers

ND PENN

The word calliper is often used interchangeably with braces or orthoses to describe external supportive devices for the leg. Generally, the term orthosis (derived from orthos meaning to straighten) should be used to describe a device applied to the external surface of the body to improve function. Leg orthoses can be divided into (a) foot orthoses such as insoles and heel wedges; (b) ankle-foot orthoses, which extend above the ankle; (c) knee-ankle-foot orthoses; and (d) hip-knee-ankle-foot orthoses. Although leg orthoses have popularly been referred to as callipers (probably based on the similarity of the construction of early callipers to the measuring instrument of the same name), the term "brace" (more commonly used in the United States) is perhaps now more appropriate and is becoming more widely used. The functions of leg orthoses are:

- to provide stability for weakened, paralysed, or unstable legs
- to relieve weight bearing
- to relieve pain
- to control deformity
- to restrict movement of the joint.

Ankle-foot orthoses

Ankle-foot orthoses are the most commonly prescribed and illustrate well the construction and functions of leg orthoses in general. There are two types: conventional orthoses of leather and metal construction and contemporary orthoses made from thermoplastics (most commonly ortholene and polypropylene).

Conventional ankle-foot orthoses consist of one or two metal uprights connected proximally by a leather calf band and distally to a mechanical ankle joint. The calf band should rest 4 cm below

133

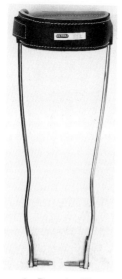

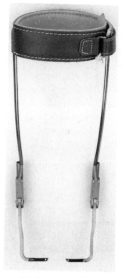

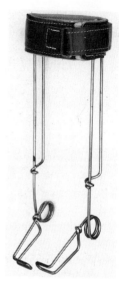

FIG 1—Round calliper

FIG 2—Square calliper with mechanical ankle joint

FIG 3—Springs at mechanical ankle joint

the tibial condyle and not impinge on the peroneal nerve below the fibular head. There should be room to insert a finger between the calf band and the leg, and the metal uprights should not press against the leg. The orthoses may be attached to the shoe by a rounded socket in the heel (which then acts as a mechanical joint, fig 1) or by a square socket which then requires a proximal mechanical ankle joint (fig 2). Both types of orthoses restrict movement in the sagittal plane. Movement can be helped, limited, or prevented by incorporating springs or stops at the joint. Stops can be preset to allow any predetermined degree of movement. Movement at the ankle joint may be helped or restricted by using springs or elastic straps across the joint (fig 3).

Contemporary orthoses—Orthotic design changed dramatically with the introduction of thermoplastics. The thermoplastic is shaped by applying a heated softened form to a plaster mould of the leg. They have the advantage of being light and having a more acceptable cosmetic appearance. Generally, plastic ankle-foot orthoses do not have mechanical joints. Movement at the ankle is achieved by flexing the orthosis, the shape of the orthosis around the lower calf determining the flexibility. By leaving more material

134

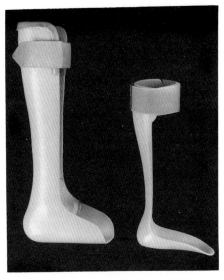

FIG 4—Thermoplastic splints, the left being the less flexible

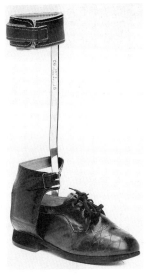

FIG 5—T strap for correcting varus deformity

anteriorly a fairly fixed orthosis can be obtained, while progressive trimming will produce a more flexible splint (fig 4). As they are in close contact with the skin their use is not advised if there is a tendency to ulceration or the legs are oedematous and prone to a change in size.

Checkpoints when examining a patient with an ankle-foot orthosis

Conventional orthosis
- calf band does not impinge on peroneal nerve
- a finger can be inserted between calf band and leg
- metal uprights are not pressing against the leg

Contemporary orthosis
- legs are not oedematous and prone to fluctuation in size
- legs are not prone to ulceration

General
- patient able to put on orthosis
- patient finds orthosis acceptable to wear
- wear and tear—for example, worn leather, cracked plastic
- uneven wear of shoe indicating inadequate support of ankle

Common indications for orthoses

Flaccid foot drop—The commonest cause of foot drop is peroneal nerve palsy, usually from pressure at the neck of the fibula. It may also be a consequence of peripheral neuropathy, nerve root lesions (sciatica), and muscular dystrophies. Whatever its cause it results in the toes dragging on the floor during walking. This may be corrected by using a thermoplastic orthosis of the required structural strength and compliance to produce sufficient dorsiflexion assistance. Alternatively a conventional orthosis with a single medial upright could be used. This could incorporate either a compression spring behind the ankle joint (producing a dorsiflexion force) or a stop, which will prevent plantar flexion.

Spastic foot drop is most commonly seen after a stroke. A spastic foot tends to adopt a position of plantar flexion with a degree of inversion and external rotation. Early physiotherapy aims to reduce spasticity and seems to prevent, minimise, or retard the degree of hypertonicity. As a result few stroke victims require mechanical support of their ankle. If patients do not respond to manual therapy physical supports may have to be considered. Boots may be all that is required to enable safe and comfortable ambulation, or when there is only mild spasticity a thermoplastic orthosis may be enough to overcome the foot drop. If further mechanical support is required the appliance should be designed to keep the foot in as functional position as possible. As muscle spasm will overcome a spring of any strength that could be tolerated by the patient their use should be avoided. Here a double bar calliper fitted with plantar flexion stops should be used together with strong well fastened shoes to prevent the heel rising out of the shoe. To help overcome inversion a T (or Y) shaped strap attached to the outside of the shoe (fig 5), covering the lateral malleolus and looped around the medial upright can be added. This pulls the lateral malleolus medially, correcting the varus position. If there is a tendency towards eversion the valgus position can be corrected with a medial strap. Inspection of the heel of the shoe for uneven wear will indicate whether sufficient support is being provided. For the patient with stroke with a knee that is so weak that bracing seems necessary, providing an above knee orthosis is unlikely to be successful. Weakness of the hip muscles together with the weight of the orthosis will prevent any considerable improvement in gait.

Patients with paraplegia resulting from a lower cord lesion—for example, lesions of the cauda equina—generally benefit from mobilisation with a leg orthoses. The higher the lesion (particularly above T10) the less likely that orthoses are to be successful. Most patients will require a metal knee-ankle-foot orthosis, though some will manage with a plastic orthosis. The usual metal orthosis consists of two metal uprights from the upper thigh to the ankle connected by rigid posterior calf and thigh bands that keep the uprights in their correct position and are closed in the front by soft fastenings. Knee locks allow flexion of the orthosis when sitting but lock to provide stability when walking. A variety of locks is available, the most common being a drop lock (ring lock) or a bail lock (Swiss lock). Stops at the ankle joint are required to prevent both plantar and dorsiflexion.

Ankle deformity—Valgus or varus deformity of the ankle (as in rheumatoid arthritis) may be corrected simply by providing appropriate footwear. If more support is required a standard single or double upright orthosis attached to a firm shoe usually provides enough ankle stability.

Pain relief—Pain in the ankle from conditions such as rheumatoid arthritis and osteoarthritis may be exacerbated by walking because of lateral deforming forces and the direct effect of weight bearing. The tendency to valgus deformity may be overcome by appropriate footwear. Alternatively an ankle-foot orthosis may have to be provided. A single or double upright orthoses with free movement at the ankle (no springs or stops being required as there is no muscle weakness) may provide enough support at the ankle to prevent painful lateral forces on the ankle. Relief of weight bearing pain at the knee may be provided by either a knee orthosis or a knee-ankle-foot orthosis.

Prescription of orthoses

Orthoses are available only on prescription from hospital specialists. The supply of orthoses to the NHS is contracted out to the private companies who tender the most competitive prices. They will send an orthotist to attend hospital clinics, who, with the consultant and physiotherapist, will assess the patient. Consideration should be paid to (*a*) what the orthosis is to achieve; (*b*) combining function with acceptable cosmetic appearance; (*c*) ensuring that the patient (and carers) know how to and are able to fit the orthosis; and (*d*) avoiding complications such as pressure sores. After fitting the orthosis the patient should be reviewed by the prescribing specialist, who can then "stabilise" the prescription for up to five years. During this period the orthosis can be repaired or replaced by the orthotist without specialist consultation. After this time, however, a new prescription has to be issued by the specialist after referral by the general practitioner. Provision and repair of leg orthoses are carried out free of charge to the patient.

Appendix

Useful reading

McHugh B, Campbell J. Below knee orthoses. *Physiotherapy* 1987;73:380–5.
Redford JB, ed. *Orthotics etcetera*. Baltimore: Williams and Wilkins, 1980.
Goodwill J. Orthotics (calipers and appliances). In: Goodwill CJ, Chamberlain MA, eds. *Rehabilitation of the physically disabled adult*. New York: Croom Helm, 1988:741.

Crutches

BARBARA E POTTER, W ANGUS WALLACE

The wooden crutches that are manufactured today bear a striking resemblance to the device used by Long John Silver. Modern day crutches, however, offer alternatives to axillary support or have a cushioned axilla pad to avoid the problems of injury to the nerves due to pressure in the axilla from the crutch. A pair of crutches allow an ambulant patient to walk and at the same time relieve weight from one or both legs by transferring weight through the arms. The crutch provides more relief of weight bearing than a standard walking stick. Ideally crutches should be light and, if possible, leave at least one hand free for activities such as opening doors. Crutches are less bulky than other devices such as walking frames but require more coordination and stability from the patient.

Crutches are needed after fractures of the legs, when partial or complete relief from weight bearing is required; to relieve pain in severe arthritis affecting one or more lower limb joints; during temporary weakness or paralysis of the leg for any reason, such as footdrop associated with a recent tibial fracture or traumatic neuropraxia, such as an anterior compartment syndrome; postoperatively for patients who have had an operation on the muscles or joints (particularly in uncemented hip replacement) when relief of weight bearing is often recommended for up to three months after the operation; for patients who have undergone amputation of a part of the leg and are waiting for their permanent prosthesis; and for patients with neurological disturbance, such as ataxia.

Types of crutch

Axilla crutches (fig 1) are the most commonly prescribed type. Those supplied by hospitals are usually made from wood and are

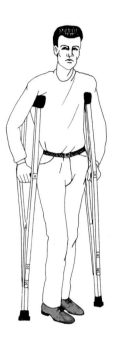

FIG 1—Axilla crutch

cheaper but slightly heavier than the commercially available metal crutches made from lightweight aluminium. The cost of wooden crutches is about £14 a pair compared with metal crutches, which cost £20 a pair. The cross piece of the crutch, which rests under the axilla, is usually padded and covered with a non-slip washable material. The hand grip can be either wooden or metal with a moulded plastic covering. The height of the hand grip and the overall height of the crutch are adjustable: in wooden crutches by means of nuts and bolts and in metal crutches by spring loaded buttons (fig 2). Wooden crutches are suitable for short term use for non-weight bearing or the early stages of partial weight bearing. When longer term use is expected metal axilla crutches are more appropriate.

Elbow crutches (fig 3) are made of aluminium tubing with an arm support of polypropylene. Some manufacturers produce an elbow crutch in which the arm support attachment to the shaft is hinged and the support is malleable, allowing adjustment to the thickness of the forearm. The hand grip is covered with moulded plastic. The overall height of the crutch below the hand grip (and on some

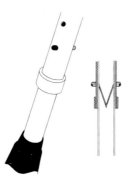

FIG 2—Spring loaded buttons

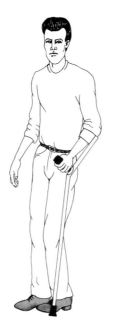

FIG 3—Elbow crutch

models above the grip) is adjustable by means of spring loaded buttons. The cost of elbow crutches is between £13 and £15 a pair. Folding elbow crutches (fig 4) are commercially available and may prove more convenient than standard elbow crutches, which can be awkward to store when not in use—for example, when the patient is travelling or in fixed seating units. Elbow crutches are

141

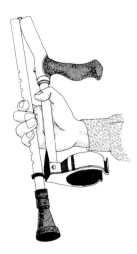

FIG 4—Folding elbow crutch (available from Cooper and Sons Ltd, Wormley, Godalming, Surrey)

suitable for partial weight relief and are not recommended for patients who cannot bear at least part of their weight on both legs. They may be indicated when it is impracticable or uncomfortable to use conventional axilla crutches—for instance, when there are rib fractures, old mastectomy, or arm injury weakness. Patients who suffer from rheumatoid arthritis or the carpal tunnel syndrome and may have a reduced hand grip power will probably find elbow crutches more convenient and easier to control.

Gutter crutches (fig 5) are similar to elbow crutches but instead of a straight crutch have a forearm gutter support with a handle set at right angles to the shaft. The gutter support is usually lined with sheepskin or a synthetic equivalent and is secured to the patient's forearm by means of Velcro straps with the hand grip covered by moulded plastic. The crutch is fully adjustable with spring loaded buttons to permit adjustment of the height between the ground and the forearm support. The telescopic forearm support has a handle that rotates through 360°. The crutch can be provided with either single or quadruped feet (inset to fig 5), quadruped feet being more applicable to patients with poor balance. The cost of gutter crutches is around £26 a pair. They have the advantage that patients are able to take weight through the forearm over a larger area of support and therefore they can be more useful for relieving weight bearing in the legs than the other types of crutches

142

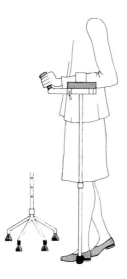

FIG 5—Gutter crutch

described. They are particularly appropriate when the range of movement in the wrist joints is either restricted or painful, such as in rheumatoid arthritis and osteoarthritis; when a forearm plaster cast is present; or when wrist splintage is required. They may also be helpful for patients with reduced hand grip strength.

A non-slip rubber ferrule is applied to the lower end of all models to prevent the crutch slipping.

Assessment of patients

Careful assessment of the patient's capability is necessary before crutches are issued or prescribed. Expenditure of energy is high when using crutches and therefore patients with cardiac and chronic chest conditions might be unsuitable. Energy expenditure when using crutches can rise by over 60% compared with the average for normal level walking.[1] As a general rule older patients should be considered for walking frames rather than crutches. Our observations are that many patients aged over 60 find the use of crutches difficult for non-weight bearing or partial weight bearing, particularly when this has to be sustained for a prolonged period or distance. Patients who may have problems in using crutches include those with multiple sclerosis, stroke, or poor vision.

143

Although patients with impaired balance generally experience difficulties when using crutches, they can be used to provide stability, particularly for patients with ataxia. The use of crutches entails the transfer of weight through the arms, and some patients may be unable to tolerate this when muscle power is reduced or joint instability is present.

Fitting the crutches

In the NHS it is usually the physiotherapist who distributes crutches on the advice or prescription of a doctor. Physiotherapists, however, are not always available, and crutches are sometimes distributed by nursing staff (or even doctors). In these cases assessment of the patients should still be made regarding their suitability for crutches and advice should be given to patients as outlined below. One crutch should not normally be issued as it may cause problems with weight distribution and possibly disturb the gait. A pair of crutches is recommended, though a combination of axillary and elbow or gutter crutch may be prescribed, depending on the needs of the individual patient. The appliance selected must be the correct size for the user and adjusted to ensure that the patient can maintain his or her normal erect posture comfortably. All adjustments should be made with the patient standing erect and wearing normal footwear. Patients should be advised to wear flat heeled shoes with non-slip soles and heels. They should be made aware of the alteration to their height that may occur if they change footwear or wear no shoes and the effect this can have on the use of their crutches. Failure to wear shoes may result in the crutches being too long and therefore pressing in the axilla, and stockinged feet may lead to slipping and therefore a fall.

The overall height of axilla crutches should be two to three finger breadths below the axilla when the crutch tip is resting on the floor 8 to 10 cm to the side of the feet and the patient is standing upright. The hand grip should be level with the distal wrist crease when the elbow is flexed to 15 or 20° with the arm resting by the side of the body. When the patient uses the axilla crutch no pressure should be transmitted from the cross piece to the axilla as this may cause pressure injuries to the posterior cord of the brachial plexus.

When elbow crutches are used the forearm support should be positioned distal to the elbow joint. The hand rest should be level with the distal wrist crease when the elbow is 15 to 20° flexed with the arm resting by the side of the body. For gutter crutches with the arm resting by the side but the elbow flexed at 90° the patient should be able to support his or her weight on the forearm and grip well enough to lift and place the crutch safely.

Problems caused by crutches

Several problems may occur for patients using crutches. Firstly, compression of the brachial plexus from incorrect use or fitting of axilla crutches. Secondly, bruising of the ribs caused by the patient gripping an axilla crutch inwards towards the chest. Thirdly, blistering or soreness of the hands due to continual pressure between hand and handle; the patient should be advised to release pressure intermittently and wear gloves or pad the handle to reduce friction. Fourthly, the carpal tunnel syndrome can occur from a poor gripping action when the palms of the hand are used incorrectly for weight bearing, and, finally, fatigue—crutches are hard work.

Care of crutches

All models require careful examination before issue, and advice should be given to the user on points that should be checked every week.

Firstly, the structure of the crutch should be inspected for signs of damage or fatigue, such as ill fitting, broken, or loose joints, cracks, or distortion. Metal and wooden crutches have been known to snap under the stress of long term use. Secondly, the wing nuts on adjustable wooden crutches should be tightened and checked for signs of wear. Thirdly, spring loaded buttons on metal crutches should be examined to ensure that all springs are working. Finally, ferrules should have a good tread. Worn ferrules may result in the crutch losing grip on wet or slippery surfaces. All patients must be advised carefully on the need for a safe ferrule and where to obtain new ferrules when they are required. The patient should be able to obtain replacement ferrules from the department where the appliance was issued. Alternatively, they may be bought from a retail outlet that supplies surgical requisites.

All hospital workers should be aware of their responsibilities under the Consumer Protection Act 1987. Because of these responsibilities crutches cannot be supplied directly to patients

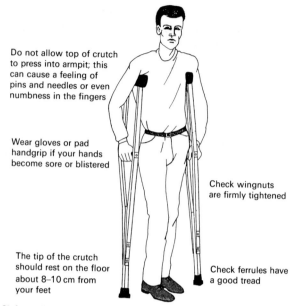

Do not allow top of crutch to press into armpit; this can cause a feeling of pins and needles or even numbness in the fingers

Wear gloves or pad handgrip if your hands become sore or blistered

Check wingnuts are firmly tightened

The tip of the crutch should rest on the floor about 8–10 cm from your feet

Check ferrules have a good tread

Slow small steps are safe, to go too fast can mean falling
Do not attempt to arise from sitting (or reverse) with crutches resting under the arms

If you experience any problems while using the crutches or with the appliance itself please seek advice from the department where you were issued with the crutches (eg fracture clinic or accident and emergency department)

PHYSIOTHERAPY SERVICES, NOTTINGHAM

FIG 6—Instruction sheet for patients

without advice being given to the patient on the use and maintenance of the crutch. Useful pointers to the implications of the act have been summarised by the Chartered Society of Physiotherapy.[2 3]

Crutch supplies are usually available in physiotherapy departments, accident and emergency departments, fracture clinics, orthopaedic wards and clinics, health centres, social services departments, and surgical appliance departments. Although it would be logical to supply all crutches from a central store through physiotherapists, this is not practical, particularly out of hours. Normally there is no charge to the patient for the loan of crutches. Some hospitals, however, demand a returnable deposit as many crutches are never returned. In Nottingham we lose up to 300 pairs of crutches a year because patients do not return them.

Warnings of possible problems or complications from using crutches should always be made to the patients together with instructions on the care of the appliance. A short teaching session on walking with crutches is necessary before the patient leaves hospital. For inpatients this will usually entail the physiotherapist teaching the patient to use the crutches around the ward as well as a trial of negotiating stairs. In the accident and emergency department, however, there are major difficulties because of the large number of patients treated and few physiotherapists are specifically employed to work in this department. A nurse normally checks that the patient can walk a few steps with the crutches but does little else. Crutches should generally be used only on even ground, and the support should be sufficient to permit swing through of the legs during walking. Special advice is required for negotiating stairs, when usually both crutches are held in one hand and the other hand is used for grasping the handrail. When crutches are used to relieve weight it is normal practice to teach the patient to ascend the stairs stepping up with the unaffected leg first. The affected leg and crutches are then transferred to the same step. Variations to this practice may occur according to the patient's diagnosis and capability. Tuition should also include the use of crutches on steps with no rail support (such as kerbs and front doors).

Some hospitals supply instructions with crutches—describing what a crutch does, how it is to be used, and the problems related to it (fig 6).

1 Waters RL, Campbell J, Thomas L, Hugos L, Davis P. Energy costs of walking in lower-extremity plaster cast. *J Bone Joint Surg [Am]* 1982;64:896–9.
2 Chartered Society of Physiotherapy. Consumer Protection Act 1987. Implications for physiotherapists. *Physiotherapy* 1988;74:175–6.
3 Chartered Society of Physiotherapy. Consumer Protection Act 1987—update. *Physiotherapy* 1988;74:530.

Appendix

Recommended reading

Reisman M, Burdett RG, Simon SR, Norkin C. Elbow movement and forces at the hand during swing-through axillary crutch gait. *Phys Ther* 1985;65:601–5.
Gillespy FC, Fisher J, Williams CS, McKay EE, Curr MCH. A physiological assessment of the rolling crutch. *Ergonomics* 1983; 26:341–7.
Walking aids. Oxford: Mary Marlborough Lodge.

Mobility aids and appliances for disabled children

KENNETH S HOLT

Aids and appliances should be provided to help immobile children whenever it would help the children and their parents and teachers. The needs of children cannot be met by scaled down versions of adult equipment. The design of equipment for children requires an understanding of their distinctive requirements. Most disabled children are afflicted early in life before the acquisition of abilities such as sitting, walking, and talking. So any equipment has to be appropriate for their stage of development and should help and not hinder their developmental progress. For example, an adult recovering from an accident can be given crutches to help walking because he or she was able to walk before the accident but a child with cerebral palsy or spina bifida can be given crutches only when he or she is developmentally ready to learn to walk. Allowances have to be made for growth and changes in body proportions. Equipment should be made according to the child's measurements; it should be supplied promptly because otherwise it may not fit when finally delivered; and it must be adjusted as growth occurs. Children like to be free and may not accept equipment that is too restrictive. Parents need to understand the purpose of any item and also how and when it should be used.

The questions to consider when prescribing a wheelchair are:

- Who will operate it? The child (with hands on large wheels or other means), or attendant (so the handles have to be of suitable height)?
- Will the chair be used outdoors? If so are the wheels suitable and the construction sturdy?

148

- Is the child restless and needing restraint (for example in athetoid cerebral palsy)?
- Does the child need postural support (such as a child at risk of scoliosis)?
- Should the chair fold (to go into a car boot or be taken on a bus)?

Buggies and wheelchairs

The "buggies" (lightweight folding frame with canvas hammock seat) that are used for most young children are suitable for disabled children. As disabled children get older larger versions are available from the district health authority wheelchair clinics (fig 1) that are suitable for moving a child from one place to another. Older children and those who spend considerable time in their chairs require something more substantial than a buggy and a wide range of pushchairs and wheelchairs is available from the disablement service centres and commercial sources. Prescribing a suitable chair is not easy. A number of questions have to be answered; measurements have to be made (fig 2); and consideration given to possible adjustments and modifications. Helpful advice can be obtained from occupational therapists and local wheelchair clinics.

Currently, the needs of most children can be met from the range

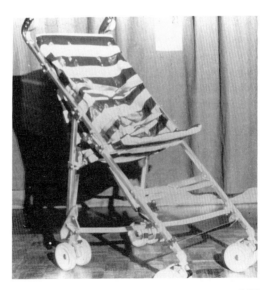

FIG 1—A major buggy

149

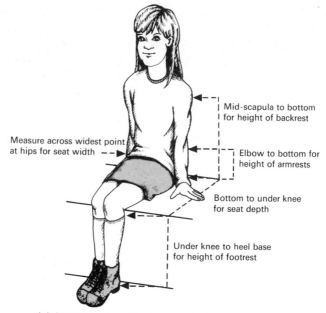

Mid-scapula to bottom for height of backrest

Measure across widest point at hips for seat width

Elbow to bottom for height of armrests

Bottom to under knee for seat depth

Under knee to heel base for height of footrest

It is important to keep hips, knees, and ankles at right angles

FIG 2—Measurements for wheelchair

Modifications and adjustments to wheelchairs (fig 3)

- Angulation of back
- Position of head rest
- Method of foot support and restraint
- Need for pommel and restraints

- Type of side supports
- Number, type, and position of cushions
- Colour

Requesting many alterations may seriously delay delivery

---

of chairs supplied by the health authority. Sometimes parents prefer to buy a chair from a commercial source, perhaps because it fulfils a distinctive need that is not covered by the other chairs or they may be the fortunate beneficiaries of charitable support. Parents buying chairs privately also have to pay for maintenance and repairs. Children who can propel their own chair require an appropriate large wheeled model, and if they participate in races and games they may want a sports model, which is strong yet lightweight. Sports models are not usually supplied by the health

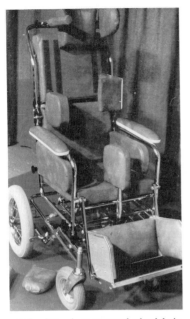

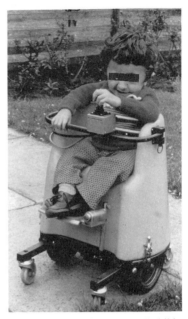

FIG 3—Attendant operated wheelchair with restraints and side supports

FIG 4—Powered chair for small child

authority unless there is a strong medical indication. A powered (battery operated) wheelchair should be considered for any disabled child who can operate the control switch and lever. The mobility that disabled children achieve and control themselves in this way is of immense benefit to their development and confidence. We have supplied such chairs to children as young as 3 years (fig 4). There are many places they can go without being on public roads. Many powered chairs are bought privately and may cost £1000 or more. A child who is so disabled as to need such a chair is usually a suitable focus for a local fund raising venture. The needs of many disabled children cannot be met by one chair: they may need two or three different ones. Consider their needs at home, at school and when travelling outdoors, and also whether their chair can be transported between home and school. When the reasons for more than one chair are set out clearly the district health authority usually sanctions their provision. Parents have to consider the maintenance of the chairs. It is advisable to:

● Provide space for storage

151

- Each week clean, check screws and fittings, oil, and check inflation of tyres (have available spanners, screwdrivers, oil can, and pump with correct end to fit the tyres)
- With a powered chair, each night recharge battery and each week top up water and check the wires (room should be well ventilated)
- Have readily available name, address, and telephone number of technical officer or private engineer.

Footwear

The footwear needs of disabled children can usually be met satisfactorily from the wide range of shoes available for all children, and unless there are particular reasons to the contrary this avenue should be explored before considering special boots and shoes. Not only is it more convenient and cheaper but preferable because the disabled child's shoes are then just like any other child's. Parents sometimes ask for special shoes in the hope that they will enable their child to walk or correct the appearance of deformed feet. Unfortunately these high expectations cannot be achieved by footwear alone. Special footwear is now available in more attractive forms and colours than previously.

A Piedro boot is often prescribed. It provides good support for the ankle, can be fitted with an ankle restraining strap, and can be laced up quickly. It is supplied in two or three different colours. The Wolfson boot (fig 5), which is a close fitting, fine leather boot fashioned on a plaster cast of the foot and worn inside another shoe or boot, provides firm yet comfortable support. Some children, especially those with hemiplegia, have feet of different sizes. Buying shoes of different sizes from an understanding shoe salesperson or by arrangement with the shoemakers may be possible. Otherwise the larger foot can be fitted and then toe inserts and heelgrips placed in the other shoe to obtain a fit on the smaller foot. Unequal leg length can be dealt with by building up the shoe on the shorter side, but this should be done only if it is recommended by doctor and therapist and is acceptable to the child and parents. Shoes can be modified in various ways, but it is better not to make any changes without the advice of a physiotherapist.

Indications for special boots or shoes are:
- Misshapen feet that cannot be fitted by ordinary footwear
- Unstable feet requiring additional support

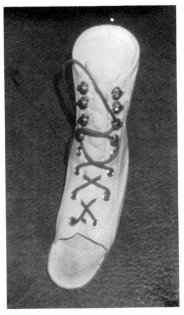

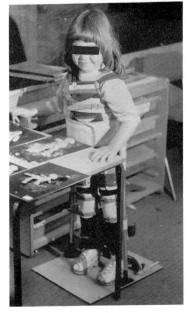

FIG 5—Wolfson boot

FIG 6—Standing frame

- Need to inhibit progression of deformity
- Need to fit or accommodate other appliances such as a short leg calliper or ankle-foot orthosis
- Need to alter pattern of gait.

Aids for standing

Early experience of standing is desirable to provide experience of being upright; to get good angulation of the femoral necks; and to give the child opportunity to use his or her hands. Standing frames, of which there are several types and sizes, are preferred to the standing boxes used in the past because they provide better control of the limbs, which also can be seen and checked easily (fig 6). The feet are fixed, and flexion of the knees (and in some cases also rotation) and the hips is controlled by broad bands in front of the chest, behind the buttocks, and in front of the knees. When knee flexion is especially troublesome gaiters may be used. Once a child is familiar with a standing frame he or she will stay in it for an hour or so—the duration of a classroom lesson. Children afflicted

153

with cerebral palsy, spina bifida, and muscular dystrophy are likely to benefit from standing frames.

Walking aids

Training disabled children to walk is a specialised task that is best carried out by a paediatric physiotherapist. The simplest walking aid is a small pram or cart or animal on wheels that the child pushes. The aid can be weighted to give stability. The rollator (a walking frame with wheels) follows the same principle (fig 7). Whenever these types of walking aids are used attention must be given to the child's posture, which may become too flexed at the hips and knees. To overcome this tendency to crouch posterior walkers, which the child pulls behind him or her, are used and they promote a more upright posture.

Some form of hand held walking aid may be considered for children with useful arms. These may be walking sticks, broom-sticks (again to encourage an upright posture), tripods, quadro-pods, and crutches. The child's condition is one of the major factors influencing the type of aid to use. For example, a child with spina bifida usually learns to use crutches quite early but one with cerebral palsy may not be able to use them until much later because of difficulties of manipulation and control. Callipers are used less often nowadays. Aversion to their heavy, cumbersome nature played some part in this but earlier therapy and better orthopaedic surgery also contributed. Short leg callipers are used to control the posture of the foot and the position of the tibia in stance when ankle-foot orthoses are not sufficient. They are used to control foot deformity and footdrop and increase stability at the ankle. Children with flail legs such as those with spina bifida, poliomyelitis, and the late stages of muscular dystrophy may need long leg callipers. In recent years attention has been given to reciprocal callipers, which have a functional role and are not just supportive and restrictive. As one leg moves forwards and begins to take weight the opposite leg of the callipers is stimulated to move forwards. Another device for a paraplegic child is the swivel walker, which depends on trunk sway to initiate the reciprocal action.

Other equipment that is useful in particular instances includes the knee cage, which controls movements at the knee, especially hyperextension, and is useful in any disorder with an unstable

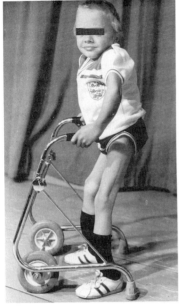

FIG 7—Rollator

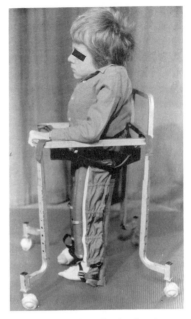

FIG 8—Inflatable orthosis, showing inflated tubes up front of leg

---

Avoid
- Baby bouncers in which the child sits in a suspended seat with his or her legs touching the floor because they encourage unsuitable movement patterns
- Baby walkers in which the child sits in a canvas seat attached to a frame with wheels because they may run away out of control.

---

knee. Children with cerebral palsy sometimes have strong spasm of their hip adductor muscles that causes their legs to cross and so impedes walking. The problem can be controlled by a thigh abduction splint, which inhibits adduction without restricting walking. An inflatable orthosis has improved the management of children with osteogenesis imperfecta (brittle bones). In the past children afflicted with this rare condition laid in bed to avoid recurrent fractures. When wrapped from mid-chest to feet in a suit composed of tubes that can be inflated with air they are given gentle, firm support and can be got to an upright position from which they can learn to walk (fig 8).

155

Acceptance of equipment

However much care is taken in the prescription of aids and appliances they are useful only if they are accepted and used by the disabled. Adults usually understand the purpose of anything provided and cooperate to get the full benefit from their equipment. Children, especially if young or retarded, do not have this ready understanding and motivation to cooperate so ways have to be found to ensure acceptance of the equipment. Concerned adults have to be informed, and thought has to be given to the design of the equipment. There are many simple and cheap ways by which equipment can be made attractive and appealing to children. Fortunately, manufacturers are realising the importance of design, colour, and even camouflage. The attitudes of parents, teachers, and therapists greatly influence children and may be the determining factor in children's acceptance or rejection of equipment. Offhand detached attitudes and overforceful persuasion are often counterproductive.

At all stages in managing disabled children attention has to be given to all the family, and this is especially so when introducing equipment. Parents may resent that their child has to wear unsightly equipment that proclaims that he or she is crippled or they may themselves not understand its purpose. All this comes when they are still deeply distressed to have a disabled child. Introducing any item of equipment requires sensitive and sometimes prolonged discussion with the parents until they fully understand its purpose, support its use, and work with you to achieve acceptance by the child.

Appendix

Further information

Disabled Living Foundation, 380–384 Harrow Road, London W9 2HU (071 289 6111). The Disabled Living Foundation will give you the address of your local disabled living centre, which will provide helpful advice on equipment for disability.
Spastics Society, 12 Park Crescent, London W1N 4EQ.
Association for Spina Bifida and Hydrocephalus, 22 Upper Woburn Place, London WC1H 0EP.
Muscular Dystrophy Group, Nattrass House, 35 Macauley Road, London SW4 0QP.
Brittle Bone Society, 112 City Road, Dundee DD2 2PW.

Ramps and rails

AF TRAVERS

About 1 in 100 members of the population of the United Kingdom uses a wheelchair[1] and many more have other disabilities. A quarter of the over 75s are housebound,[2] in some cases for lack of a simple means of crossing their own doorsteps. Others, though able to get out of the house, cannot travel easily or enter other buildings. Ramps empower disabled people by providing access to their homes, other buildings, and vehicles. Rails are the simplest of housing adaptations and can also do much to ease mobility.

Ramps

A simple dropped kerb at road crossing points eases the passage of anyone in a wheelchair. Sheltered housing complexes are sometimes designed with continuous dropped kerbs throughout. The gradient of a dropped kerb should not exceed 1 in 10.

Materials

Ramps may be portable or fixed. A wide variety of commercially available ramps complement the construction by local authorities of permanent ramps at the dwellings of disabled people. Construction materials include aluminium, which is strong for its weight and durable; glass reinforced plastic, which is self coloured, easy to clean, resists rust, rot, and corrosion without maintenance and has a high strength to weight ratio; and wood, which is cheap, quick to use, and suitable for immediate temporary use. It should be preservative treated to prevent rot. Sometimes expanded metal mesh is used as the surface material; this prevents snow and rain from reducing the friction between the wheels of the chair and the surface of the ramp. Such ramps should have solid ends to help the user to start rising.

157

Surfaces

The surface of the ramp should be non-slip, and various safety treads are available. Some portable ramps have non-slip material on the underside of their ends to prevent slippage. Simple wooden ramps can be surfaced with rubber (fig 1). Concrete can be patterned or brushed to give a slip resistant surface.[3] Outdoor ramps may be crowned to drain off rain. Solid rubber ramps have non-slip "stepped" surfaces suitable for mounting kerbs. These measure 30 × 30 cm and are about 8 cm high at their raised ends, but they have an interlocking device on the side so that any width of ramp can be built up by adding extra sections. They are heavy but have a high strength to weight ratio and are even used by some fire brigades. Their small size makes them easy to stow.

Design

Modular ramp systems (fig 2) can incorporate straight runs, dogs leg sections (for turning the ramp through 180°), corners, inclines, and levels linked together according to access and the level of the entrance. Both left and right handed versions are available and cost about £160 a metre. These are usually permanent fixtures but can sometimes be removed and resited. Unlike permanent concrete ramps they do not interfere with ventilation or the damp course.

The gradient of a ramp should not exceed 1 in 12 (about 5°) and should ideally be up to 1 in 20 to allow for independent wheelchair users. With a strong carer and a light wheelchair and passenger combination a gradient of 1 in 8 may sometimes be manageable where space is limited, though this is not recommended. Any crossfall or camber should not exceed 1 in 100 or a chair may veer out of control.

Safety

The top of a permanent or semipermanent metal ramp should be bolted to the underlying surface. The edges of the ramp should be raised 7·5 cm for safety (fig 1), and some glass fibre ramps have contrast coloured edges, which are especially useful for the partially sighted. The leading edge should taper to ground level to facilitate the ascent of the wheelchair.

Handrails should be provided for the use of ambulant disabled people, at least along the outside edge and preferably at both sides of the ramp at a height of 1 metre. If the ramp is more than 2

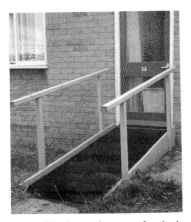 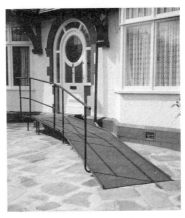

FIG 1—Simple wooden ramp for single step approach

FIG 2—Individually designed modular ramp and platform system. (Reproduced courtesy of Rolac Ltd)

metres wide a central handrail can be used. These rails can be made of preservative treated wood or metal. Another feature of ramped entrances that should be provided for the ambulant disabled is simultaneous step access, with handrails, as ramped surfaces can be difficult to ascend for those who are not able bodied.

Rest platforms (preferably 180 cm × 180 cm) should be provided at the top of the ramp, and this area should not be encroached on by outwardly opening doors. The entrance door at the top of the ramp should give an opening width of at least 80 cm. There should also be rest platforms at least every 6 metres along the ramp. The ramp itself should be at least 1 metre wide, although in general domestic ramps need not be as wide as those in public buildings. The area at the bottom of the ramp should be level, free of gravel and loose material, and should provide room for safe manoeuvring of the wheelchair.

Stepped ramps consist of long sloping treads at a gradient of 1 in 12 interspersed with short (5–10 cm) risers, up which the wheelchair can be pushed as if up a shallow kerb. Platform steps are similar but have level resting platforms between each riser. Such an arrangement is used where there is not enough room for a full length ramp of the correct gradient, but it is of no use for a wheelchair user who has to climb the ramp alone. These stepped arrangements are far from ideal and are not mentioned in British Standards.

159

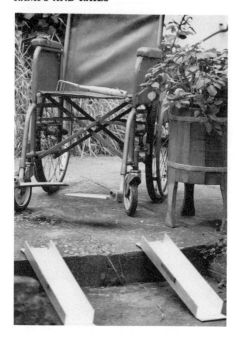

FIG 3—Portable single step channelling ramps. (Reproduced courtesy of Mobility Engineering Design Ltd)

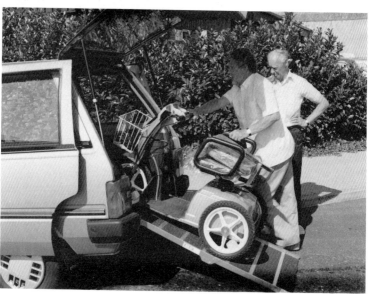

FIG 4—Portable vehicle ramp for unoccupied chairs, etc. (Reproduced courtesy of Rolac Ltd)

160

Portable ramps

Portable ramps are useful for active disabled people who visit areas outside the home for work and recreation. Raised thresholds caused by patio door casings and weather sills can be overcome by internal wooden ramps or bridge plates.

Channelling ramps are one type of portable ramp in which the nearside and offside sets of wheels run in separate channels between the two levels to be negotiated (fig 3). In some versions the inside parapets are missing to enable wheelchairs with low ground clearance to clear the ramps. Each ramp needs to be 13 cm wide to accommodate the offset wheels of some chairs. They are usually made of lightweight aluminium and fold up so that they are portable and can be carried in a pouch on the back of the wheelchair or in a vehicle. Some have crossbars between the two channels that lock the two halves of the ramp together for stability. Some are strong enough to convey powered invalid cars. Channelling ramps can be used only by competent attendants as they need to walk between the channels pushing the chair to shoulder height, and when descending they must first go down the steps backwards while controlling the chair. Many other portable ramps of various strengths are available. They are generally lightweight with raised edges and safe surfaces. Sometimes they can be linked together to form long sections or may be of fixed length but telescope or fold down for storage or transportation. They cost about £150 a metre.

Folding ramps are mounted in wall brackets but swing across the entrance and down into their operating positions when required. They are suitable for awkward entrances.

Vehicle ramps

Vehicle ramps are available from many manufacturers (fig 4). Various sizes suit most minibuses and estate cars up to a floor height of about 60 cm. They are quick and cheap alternatives to hydraulic or electric tail lifts and freestanding hydraulic collapsible wheelchair lifts. Some have vertical pivots that open like a door for escaping in an emergency, cleaning, or using the passenger step. Others are mounted at either rear or side doors of the vehicle. Some may be stowed under the floor and can be slid out in seconds; others are stowed vertically inside the rear doors. Vehicle ramps can be free standing, "hook on," or be permanently fixed inside the

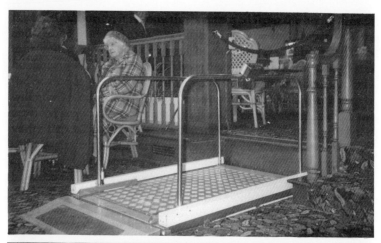

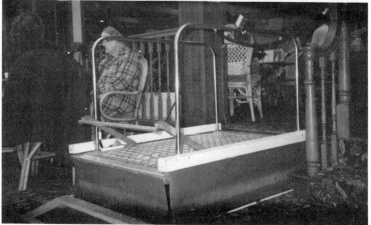

FIG 5—Short rise lift with ramp access: (*top*) descended position; (*bottom*) ascended position

back of the vehicle. They may have a leg support system for heavy wheelchair and passenger combinations. Prices range from £250 for a pair of vehicle channelling ramps to £700 for a substantial minibus ramp.

All new "purpose built taxis" now have to be wheelchair accessible with ramps and grab handles, wide opening doors, collapsible back seats, and seat belts for the wheelchair user.[1] Older taxis can be converted to this standard.

British Rail's *Station Design Guide for Disabled Customers* lays down guidelines for the construction of ramps in accordance with the features listed above.

Short rise lifts

Short rise lifts serve the same function as fixed ramps where space is limited or disability too great for a ramp to be used (fig 5). Like ramps they are covered by British Standards. The wheelchair is wheeled on to a platform which, at the touch of a button, moves between two levels. If the mechanism fails it is possible to raise and lower the lift by hand. The upper and lower platforms have safety gates and guard rails. Sometimes there is a short access ramp to the lower platform or the lift mechanism is sunk into a pit below the lower landing, and access is therefore level. The lift platform should have a non-slip finish. Their prices range from £1500 to £6000.

Grab rails and handrails

Staircase handrails should be continuous and should extend 30 cm beyond the steps at top and bottom. Ideally they should be colour contrasted against the background. The ends of the rail should be returned to the wall to show a visually handicapped user that the rail has finished and to prevent the open end from catching the user's clothing and causing an accident. The handrail should be 85 cm higher than the start of each tread and 1 metre higher than the floor and landing levels. There should be a space of 4·5 cm wide between the rail and the wall, and the rail should be 4·5–5·0 cm in diameter, but other profiles are acceptable if they give the same degree of hand grip. A Stair Aid is a rectangular handle that is fixed in a grooved runner the length of the flight of stairs and grasped by the user and slid up or down as appropriate. If the user starts to trip and thus presses down on the device it will automatically lock in position.

Door handles should be set about 104 cm above floor level and lever door handles are preferred to knobs. One way to make it easier for a wheelchair user to close an away opening door is to fix either a full width closing bar or a large D shaped handle to the back of the door nearer to the hinges than to the opening edge. A D handle can also be fixed to the door frame to give a wheelchair occupant something to hang on to while unlocking the door.[3]

Bathroom rails—In the toilet and bathroom it is recommended

163

that rails are placed horizontally the full width of the back of the door, parallel with the side of the toilet, vertically adjacent to the wash basin, and on the wall behind the toilet. Fixed rails should never be positioned so as to prevent wheelchair access alongside the toilet pan. Double foldaway rails, which are available in different lengths, either single or in pairs either side, are most useful when placed parallel to the side of the toilet, especially where both able bodied and disabled people share the use of the lavatory. Drop down legs are available to give extra support to such rails, which can also be handy alongside the bed, in the kitchen, and across the top of the stairs. A large backplate enables even spread of the load.

Anchor poles, which stretch vertically from floor to ceiling, can be useful when placed in strategic positions away from wall based supports.

Grab rails are supplied by several manufacturers and come in various shapes, lengths, colours, materials, and finishes. Their diameter is usually 3–4 cm, and their loadbearing capacity is about 150 kg. Figure 6 shows a bright, contrast coloured, plastic coated grab rail used as part of a series of similar rails to enable descent from house to garden for the ambulant disabled. Grab rails are particularly useful at thresholds and entrances. The precise positioning, number, and type of grab rails depends on the layout of the home and on the user's disabilities. Determining the basic dimensions depends on age, sex, and anthropometric criteria.[4] Grab rails need not be straight; they can be angled at 45° if the fixing point would otherwise restrict grip—for example, by being too near a door jamb. Angled shapes give added leverage. Straight grab rails can be arranged in series with minimum intermediate gaps along the wall of a corridor or hall.

Materials—Stainless steel grab bars are easy to clean but cold to touch, do not always provide a smooth grip, and can look institutional. They are, therefore, often coated with coloured nylon or epoxy resin, the last providing a grip even with soapy hands. Chrome rails can, however, have a knurled finish to provide a firmer grip. Polystyrene rails are warm to touch and ridged for gripping. Wooden rails for outdoor use look attractive but can easily fall into disrepair. Grab rails cost about £5–£30.

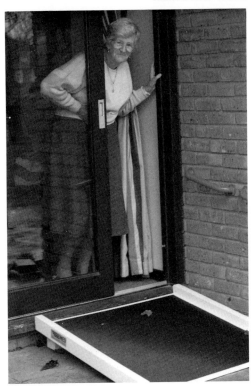

FIG 6—Grab rail at entrance. (Reproduced courtesy of Mobility Engineering Design Ltd)

Funding

Sources of funding for ramps and rails depend on whether the property concerned is owned by the local authority or is private. Funding is also governed by the cost of the items required, and arrangements vary between different local authorities. The community occupational therapist (based at the local social services department) makes the initial assessment of need.[5] Minor adaptations (those costing under £500) are dealt with and budgeted for by social services for private property and by the housing department for council homes, the actual work usually being contracted out privately. For major structural adaptations costing over £500–£1000—for example, concrete ramps—council tenants receive a grant or partial grant from the department of environmental health, whereas those in privately owned property may receive a grant after undergoing a means test. The means test is applied to

165

everyone living in the household. Those who "fail" the means test and pay for the adaptation themselves will have the payment they have made held in their favour should the need arise for an application to be made for a second adaptation in the future. Again, the actual work is contracted out privately. For a publicly used building, such as a church, the council may provide half the cost of a ramp, but local arrangements vary. No value added tax is payable on privately bought ramps if the user is chronically sick or disabled.

Ramps and rails provide the keys to accessibility to many disabled people. Their value seems obvious, but evaluation of different types has been scarce. Sweeney *et al* studied several portable ramps available in the United Kingdom and found that subjects' preferences depended on whether they propelled themselves or were pushed by an attendant, the type of wheelchair, the visual ability of user and attendant and their social needs.[6] They advised individual testing by each user of any ramp in the environment in which it would be used before purchase. A visit to the nearest disabled living centre should ensure that the most appropriate purchase is made.

1 London Taxis International. *Purpose built taxis.* Coventry: London Taxis International, 1990.
2 Hall RGP, Channing DM. Age, pattern of consultation, and functional disability in elderly patients in one general practice. *BMJ* 1990;**301**:424–8.
3 Jay P. *Coping with disability.* 2nd ed. London: The Disabled Living Foundation, 1984.
4 Health and Comfort. *Capital range grab rails and support systems.* Westbury: Health and Comfort, 1990.
5 Mandelstam M. *How to get equipment for disability.* London: Jessica Kingsley, 1990.
6 Sweeney GM, Clarke AK, Harrison RA, Bulstrode SJ. An evaluation of portable ramps. *British Journal of Occupational Therapy* 1989;**52**:473–5.

Appendix

Further reading

British Standards Institution. *Code of practice for the design of housing for the convenience of disabled people.* London: BSI, 1978. (BS5619.)
British Standards Institution. *Code of practice for access for the disabled to buildings.* London: BSI, 1979. (BS5810.)
The Royal Association for Disability and Rehabilitation. *Access data sheets Nos 1–7.* London: RADAR.
Thorpe S. *Access design sheet No 1. Ramps.* London: Centre for Accessible Environments.

Department of Environment and Welsh Office. *Building regulations 1985. Approved document part M. Access for disabled people.* London: HMSO, 1985.

Department of Architecture and Design (BRB). *Station design guide for disabled customers.* London: British Railways Board, 1989.

British Standards Institution. *Code of practice for lifts and service lifts.* London: BSI, 1986 (BS5655).

British Standards Institution. *Code of practice for the design of powered homelifts.* London: BSI, 1980. (BS5900.)

Goodwill CJ, Chamberlain MA. *Rehabilitation of the physically disabled adult.* London: Croom Helm, 1988.

Stairlifts

JANET STOWE

Most houses have the bedrooms, bathroom, and toilet on the first floor or higher. A stairlift enables a person who has problems climbing stairs to reach upper parts of the house with less difficulty.

What is a stairlift?

A stairlift is a device that transports a person up and down stairs, either sitting on a seat or standing on a platform; most have a seat. The electrically driven motor is usually under the seat on a platform. The platform rides up and down on a track that is superficially mounted on to the staircase itself. Stairlifts are as compact as possible, often folding to take up as little as 25 cm of the stair width. They are usually operated by a rocker or toggle switch by either user or carer (fig 1).

There are over 20 different stairlifts currently available in the United Kingdom, most of which go up and down a straight staircase and cost about £1500. A few go round corners and this entails more complicated engineering, which is reflected in the cost—upwards of £3000. Occasionally where there is a half turn in the landing and a further two or three steps an adaptation can be made to use a straight stairlift. The life expectancy of a stairlift can be over 20 years. It is an expensive piece of equipment that also takes up quite a lot of space at the top and bottom of the stairs and on the staircase itself.

There are several ways in which people with difficulties in climbing stairs tackle this problem. Some go up and down on their bottoms—a safe procedure if not a little uncomfortable—others may go up and down on all fours, descending backwards. As long as the patient (and carer) is happy to manage in this way there is

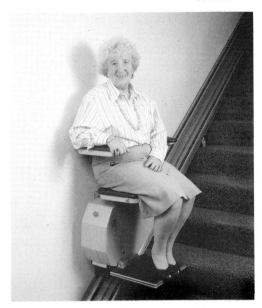

FIG 1—Stairlift in use

usually no need or reason to install a stairlift. There are, however, cheaper alternatives to installing a stairlift: stair rails on each side of the staircase and strategically placed grab handles are often sufficient to enable disabled people to use stairs more easily. These may be at the top and bottom of the stairs and, where relevant, on a bend in the staircase. They can be provided by the social services department.

If a wheelchair is to be used a through floor lift may be more suitable as fire regulations need to be considered. There has to be a way of ensuring that the disabled person is not stranded upstairs. A through floor lift transports a patient in a wheelchair on a seat in the lift, or standing from one floor to another through a trap in the ceiling. The lift usually runs on two tracks fitted to the wall, and the lift is kept in the upper floor when not in use, leaving just the tracks in view.

Why install a stairlift?

Usually all the family sleep on the same floor without one member of the family alone downstairs. It often helps those caring for a disabled person (especially those suffering from multiple

169

sclerosis or stroke) to be nearby and within earshot when help is needed during the night. To convert a living room into a bedroom with the possible addition of a commode is in most households inconvenient and unacceptable. Patients using stairlifts are usually delighted to be able to use the house normally and not be seen as a cause of disruption and loss of living space. They may also be thrilled at the new found ability to go up and down stairs with comparative ease. Stairlifts rarely break down and if they do so there is usually an established system to repair them speedily as it is recognised that a non-working stairlift means a stranded user.

Who needs a stairlift?

Many thousands of people who would otherwise be unable to use stairs use stairlifts. Those with a wide range of disabilities and difficulties such as arthritis, stroke, and coronary disease may benefit. Sometimes those with progressive disease, such as multiple sclerosis, are supplied with stairlifts, especially in the early stages. Otherwise through floor lifts are supplied in anticipation of transporting a wheelchair from ground floor to first floor (fig 2).

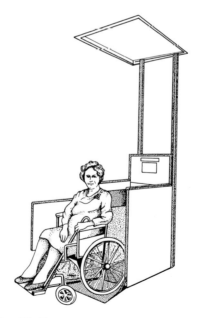

FIG 2—Through floor lift (Reproduced courtesy of Sunrise Medical Ltd)

Handicapped children grow and become heavy for parents to carry up and down stairs. Depending on the disability either a stairlift or lift can be supplied.

How to get a stairlift for your patient

Doctors should consider aids and equipment whenever they have patients who have difficulty climbing the stairs. Stairlifts can be provided by the local authority social services department, which has a legal responsibility to provide them when necessary. Patients may, however, be means tested. When there are cash shortages it is not uncommon for provision of stairlifts to be withheld or simply not allowed. This may mean that discharge from hospital is delayed. Without stairlifts managing disabled people at home may place extra strain on carers. As there are so many variations across the country in the method of providing stairlifts the time factor varies considerably from area to area between the assessment for a stairlift and the actual provision and installation. It may vary from two weeks to two years. This of course may lead to much anger and frustration by the patient and carers, who are already in a stressful situation and being stretched to their limit. Often many different staff are concerned, each responsible for a different aspect of provision and each giving different advice and information, leaving the patient and carers most confused. Nation wide we need key workers to whom people could relate and who could take overall responsibility for providing such equipment and answer all questions and queries, thus relieving the patients and carers of the stresses of conflicting information and advice.

The local social services department usually has an occupational therapist, who will visit the home and carry out an initial assessment of the patient's needs. This assessment is often carried out with a social services engineer. Together they can accurately assess the patient, the carers, and the home so that the most suitable stairlift is provided. The department of environmental health is usually involved in the acquisition of a stairlift (unless it is being bought privately) as the environmental health officer assesses patients for grants towards the cost of providing a stairlift. All areas of Britain differ in their financing of stairlifts. It would be sensble if all local authorities operated a uniform funding system. When a stairlift is no longer needed, depending on the practice of the local authority, it is sometimes removed from the home, stored, and reused elsewhere. Other times it may be the property of the user and the family to dispose of themselves. Stairlifts may be bought privately but even in these cases it is advisable first to seek the advice of the local social services occupational therapist, who will give an informed and unbiased opinion. The stairlift has to be serviced regularly to ensure its safety. The responsibility for this varies depending on local arrangements.

Assessing a patient for a stairlift is a specialised skill (fig 3): not only does the patient's physical disability, shape, and size need to be assessed to determine the dimensions of the seat and the height of the footrest but also the prognosis of the disease, the patient's psychological state, and his or her ability to follow instructions must be established. In addition, the stairlift should be matched to the house in many aspects including access at the top and bottom of stairs and needs of other people living in the house. If the patient, carers, and home are correctly assessed the installation of a

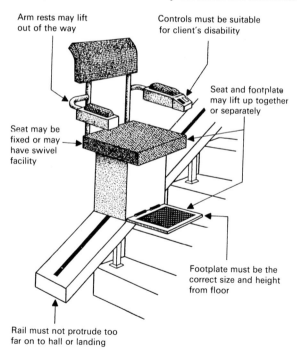

FIG 3—Some points to consider when selecting a stairlift. (Reproduced courtesy of Sunrise Medical Ltd)

stairlift should make life easier and happier for all. There should be no problems to either patient or carer unless of course the medical conditions of either person should alter. In this case, the occupational therapist should be contacted again for reassessment. It may be that guidance on lifting and manoeuvring is all that is required.

If a patient has problems of mobility in the home and a stairlift would possibly be a helpful solution there are several ways of contacting the relevant staff, depending on the facilities of the district. Ideally, the occupational therapist at the patient's local social services office will be the person to contact. The therapist can be contacted directly by the general practitioner. If there is no such facility at the social services office then try the occupational therapy department in the local general hospital, the main social services office, or the department of environmental health. In areas where there is a disabled living centre (of which there are 30 around the country) it is advisable to visit a centre where the patient and carers can try out a variety of stairlifts to discover preferences in design. The occupational therapist will be able to tell you where the nearest centre is.

I thank Ruth Whittaker, of Leeds Social Services, for her help and Glynis Cooper and Barbara Dibb for their secretarial help.

Appendix

Useful addresses

Disabled Living Foundation, 380–384 Harrow Road, London W9 2HU (071 289 6111). The Disabled Living Foundation will provide the address of your local Disabled Living Centre, which provides helpful advice on equipment for disability.

Royal Association for Disability and Rehabilitation, 25 Mortimer Street, London W1 (071 637 5400).

College of Occupational Therapy, 6–8 Marshalsea Road, Southwark, London SE1 1HL (071 357 6480).

Further reading

Stowe J. How to give your home a lift. *Care Weekly* 1988 Oct 7:28.

Goodwill CJ, Chamberlain MA, eds. *Rehabilitation of the physically disabled adult.* London: Croom Helm, 1988.

Stowe J. *Guide to the selection of the stairlifts.* Available from Rheumatology and Rehabilitation Research Unit, 36 Clarendon Road, Leeds LS2 9NZ. (£3.00).

British Standards Institution. *Specification for powered stairlifts.* Leeds: BSI, 1979. (BS5776.)

Walking frames

GRAHAM MULLEY

The first walking frame was designed and made in 1924 by a 12 year old Cincinnati boy, Charles Williams.[1] His aunt had broken her hip and after treatment could move around her hospital room only by standing at the back of her armchair and pushing it in front of her. Charles fashioned a simple wooden walking frame that enabled his aunt to walk with more ease and confidence. The local hospital was impressed with his design and made several metal frames out of gas piping. In the 1950s aluminium frames were produced, and subsequently many modifications and additions were developed. The frame is now one of the most widely used walking aids in the world.

There are over 40 types of walking frame available in Britain. The generalist does not need to know about them all but might be interested in the basic principles of use and want to learn about their advantages and disadvantages, how to obtain them, and how to inspect them for safety.

Who uses walking frames

Frames encourage safer ambulation and independence in frail elderly people. About 85% of those using them are over 65, their mean age being 75. Loss of confidence and deteriorating balance are the main symptoms affecting those who use frames, most users suffering from arthritis, hip fracture, or stroke. Walking frames ease pain by taking some of the body's weight through the arms; they also provide confidence and stability.

Types of frame

Simple frames are used in the home; larger specialised frames are more commonly found in hospitals and rehabilitation units.

174

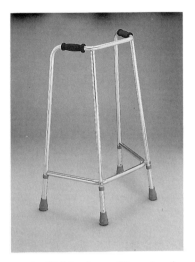

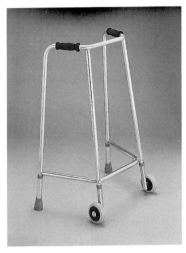

FIG 1—Walking frame. (Reproduced courtesy of Days Medical Aids Ltd)

FIG 2—Wheeled frame. (Reproduced courtesy of Days Medical Aids Ltd)

Walking frames can be of fixed or variable heights. Some have wheels, some are folding. The basic four legged, three sided walking frame is the most commonly used (fig 1), being provided to three quarters of users outside the hospital. These frames are often known as Zimmer frames (after one of the manufacturers of these aids). They are sometimes called pulpit frames. This term, however, can be used for different types of frame: as it is unhelpful and may cause confusion it should perhaps be abandoned. Ideally, patients should not stoop when standing with the frame but hold it with the elbows flexed to about 15–20°. They should have well fitted footwear, not go barefoot or wear loose slippers. To use it correctly the patient lifts the frame, puts it down in front without overstretching, takes two even steps into the frame, and stops. He or she then lifts the frame again and repeats the process. These frames are stable but inevitably produce an abnormal, halting gait. They do not allow for the normal rotation of the trunk that occurs in walking. A less abnormal pattern is produced by wheeled frames.

Wheeled frames (fig 2) have two wheels or castors at the front. They can therefore be pushed along rather than having to be lifted. Ambulation is not only smoother and faster but it requires less effort. These frames are preferred for those whose painful

175

shoulders make lifting the frame difficult; those with mild retropulsion; and mentally infirm patients with mobility problems. They are sometimes helpful in parkinsonism. Many parkinsonian patients have difficulty initiating movement; they are therefore hindered by the stop-start-stop sequence of a walking frame. The wheeled frame helps mobility but care must be taken with those who have festinant gait; once underway, they may have difficulty stopping. Frames with small wheels do not run well over carpets, but wheels of a larger diameter do run more freely. Another type of wheeled frame is a rollator (fig 3). Here again the terminology can be confusing. Some people call any wheeled frame a rollator; I have limited the term to a large stable frame that usually has handles of adjustable height. There are two wheels at the front and two rubber ferrules (or sometimes two more wheels) at the back. Some have brakes. This frame may be useful for patients with retropulsion, for some parkinsonian patients, and for children with cerebral palsy. It has a large turning circle and is therefore difficult to manoeuvre.

Tri-wheeled walkers (or delta frames) (fig 4) are mobile triangular folding frames with a single front castor and two rear wheels, which usually have brakes. Two types of brakes are available: cable brakes and spring loaded brakes that work by bearing weight on the hand grips. The height and angle of the handles can be adjusted. These frames are easier to steer than walking frames and have a small turning circle. They are, however, more unstable and difficult to use. Modified tri-wheeled walkers may be helpful in improving the mobility of some patients who are disabled by emphysema.[2] By leaning forwards on to a wheeled frame a third of the body weight can be taken through the aid and patients find that they can double their walking distance. As with all wheeled frames, they are useful only over smooth, level terrain.

The alpha frame (fig 5) is a two sided frame that can also be folded flat. This is useful for patients wanting to use cars or public transport. They are not as wide as standard walking frames and are therefore preferable when there are narrow doorways. The hands are held close together, however, when holding the handles and the patient may feel less confident when using this frame. If the frame is not well maintained it sometimes fails to lock open when in use and this can be hazardous.

The reciprocal frame (fig 6) is like a short, hinged clothes horse. The idea is to allow a normal reciprocal walking pattern—as the

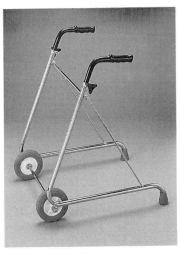

FIG 3—Rollator. (Reproduced courtesy of Days Medical Aids Ltd)

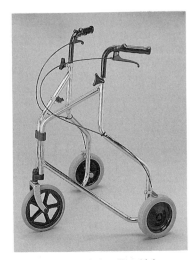

FIG 4—Tri-wheeled walker (delta frame). (Reproduced courtesy of Days Medical Aids Ltd)

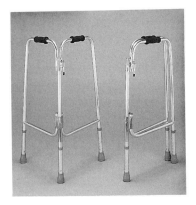

FIG 5—Folding frame (alpha frame). (Reproduced courtesy of Days Medical Aids Ltd)

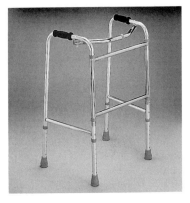

FIG 6—Reciprocal frame. (Reproduced courtesy of Days Medical Aids Ltd)

left leg advances so does the right arm. In practice, patients have difficulties learning how to use it and the frame is awkward in the home. These frames are not popular with elderly patients.

The gutter frame (fig 7) is a larger mobility aid that allows the patient to take support through the forearms. This is particularly useful when the hands are painful or deformed or when the patient

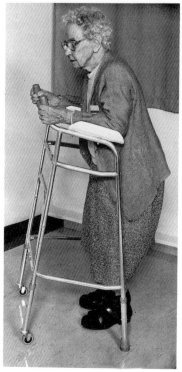 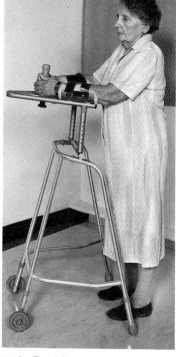

FIG 7—Gutter frame   FIG 8—Bond frame

requires maximum weight relief or support. Gutter frames have two castors at the front and can therefore be pushed along. As they are big and lack manoeuvrability they are not often used in the home.

The Bond frame (fig 8) can be an adjunct to stroke rehabilitation. The arms are placed in an armrest trough and the fingers of both hands are interlocked round a central handgrip. There are two small front wheels. This frame gives support, maintains symmetry, and keeps the arms in the extended anti-spastic position.

Modifications to walking frames

There are other modifications and additions to frames that may be helpful in individual cases. A bandage tied across the lower side bars will discourage the patient from walking too far into the

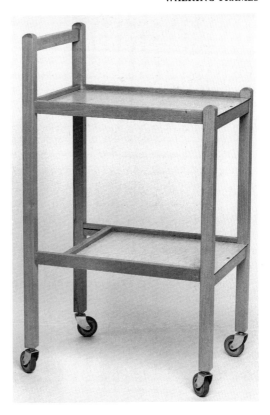

FIG 9—Trolley

frame, which can cause instability. Patients with stammering gait
(gait apraxia) may benefit from the addition of flippers fixed low
down on the rear legs and projecting into the centre of the frame.
The patient has to step over these, and using this adaptation may
help overcome the tendency of the feet to stick to the floor.[3]

Baskets can be fitted on to the front of a frame. Many patients,
however, prefer a trolley (fig 9), which allows them, for example, to
push food and utensils from the kitchen to the sitting room as well
as giving them support. Other additions include seats, trays,
shopping bags, and expanded handles for arthritic patients.

Frames are used not only for ambulation. Other uses have been
as plant stands, as a television aerial (apparently they give good
reception), and as a clothes horse to dry "smalls."

Provision of frames and education in their use

The current procedures for providing frames are variable. In a survey of 203 users of walking frames in the east Midlands, Mayfield found that frames were obtained from social services, the Red Cross, hospitals, general practitioners, and district nurses.[4] In some districts frames are provided by community physiotherapists. About 3% of patients buy their frames privately.

Physiotherapists consider it important that patients are assessed to determine whether a frame is necessary—other aids or techniques may be more appropriate. Patients should be taught how to get up from a chair and stand with a frame. Instead of pushing down on to the chair arms and holding the frame once a standing position has been adopted some patients attempt to pull themselves up out of the chair on to the frame. This is potentially dangerous: though frames are broad based they can be pulled over, causing the patient to fall backwards. One should not be too dogmatic as some patients do seem to get up better by leaning forward and pushing themselves up from their frame. Training should also include advice on walking through doorways, turning, and moving backwards and sideways.

Practical problems and solutions

Environmental limitations—Standard walking frames cannot be used on stairs (though there are specialised frames for this purpose). Users who go upstairs to bed or to the toilet will therefore require two frames—one for upstairs, the other for downstairs—and may need handrails on both sides of the stairs. Frames are unsafe on uneven terrain and care should be taken on inclines (including ramps). Frames are often too large to manoeuvre in small rooms. Some patients prefer to get around by holding on to strategically placed furniture. It is difficult to negotiate doorways, and the frame may have to be used sideways. Frames occupy a lot of space; they are rarely allowed on buses or in ambulances. Folding frames should be considered when these circumstances arise.

Effects on gait and posture—Frames offer stability but severely restrict walking speed: it is not surprising that only a third of those with frames at home use them outside. Sometimes slowing down a patient can be helpful: some walk too quickly and are at risk of falling forwards. For parkinsonian patients, who tend to assume a flexed posture, the use of two sticks may encourage a better pattern of gait.

Safety—One in eight frames shows signs of damage or has been repaired in the past. Those who issue frames must ensure that they are free from defects, safe, and clean. Assessment of disabled patients is not complete until their aids and appliances have been inspected. Important points to look out for are:

- Signs of bending, deformation, or fracture: a quarter of patients have fallen or nearly fallen while using their frames, and if the user falls on the frame the light alloy will fatigue. It may subsequently break, causing the patient to fall again
- Protruding screws that can scratch the patient or furniture and loose or missing screws that weaken the joints of the frame
- Handgrips that have become cracked, split, or loose. In one survey one in five users complained of handgrips that slipped while in use[5]
- Hard plastic handgrips that may press on the hypothenar eminences causing ulnar nerve palsies.[6] Consider padding the handles if the patient is transmitting a lot of weight through the frame over a long period.
- That rubber tips are fitted and that they have not become worn. If you find faults with a frame contact the issuing authority.

The future

Ideally, every patient should be carefully assessed by a physiotherapist before being given a frame. If walking frames were available only from physiotherapists safety would improve, provision of frames would be more appropriate, and patients would receive proper training in their use.

I am grateful to my physiotherapist colleagues, Rosemary Taylor, Rachel Kendall, Julie Isaac, and Janet Viner, for their helpful advice.

1 Dobrin L. Origin and evolution of the walkerette. *Mount Sinai J Med* 1980;47:172–4.
2 Grant BJB, Capel LH. Walking aid for pulmonary emphysema. *Lancet* 1972;ii:1125–7.
3 Wright WB. Stammering gait. *Age Ageing* 1979;8:8–12.
4 Mayfield W. A survey of walking frame issue and use. Loughborough University of Technology: Institute for Consumer Ergonomics, 1984.
5 London Borough of Hillingdon. *Domiciliary services evaluation. II. Five types of aid in common use.* London: Social Services Research, 1976.
6 Reid RI, Ashby NA. Ulnar nerve palsy and walking frames. *Br Med J* 1982;285:778.

Index